COOK
COUNTY
ICU

COOK
COUNTY
ICU

30 Years of Unforgettable
Patients and Odd Cases

CORY FRANKLIN, MD

ACADEMY

CHICAGO

Published by Academy Chicago Publishers
An imprint of Chicago Review Press Incorporated
814 North Franklin Street
Chicago, Illinois 60610
ISBN 978-0-89733-925-4

Sections of this book have previously appeared in the *Chicago Tribune*: chapter 6 as "Making Assumptions," February 5, 2014; a portion of chapter 7 as "When a White Man Goes to a Black Man's Funeral," September 12, 2014; portions of chapter 14 as "One Enchanted Moment," June 14, 1996, and "Elvis Has Definitely Left the Building," January 11, 2015; and a portion of chapter 18 as "Caring for the Notorious Patient," June 13, 2013. Other sections have appeared in *Chicago Life Magazine*: chapter 20 as "Yule Sample," December 9, 2009; and chapter 24 as "Health Without Wealth," December 7, 2008.

Library of Congress Cataloging-in-Publication Data
Franklin, Cory M.
    Cook County ICU: 30 years of unforgettable patients and odd cases / Cory Franklin, MD.
        pages cm
    ISBN 978-0-89733-925-4
    1. John H. Stroger, Jr., Hospital of Cook County (Chicago, Ill.) 2. Intensive care units—Illinois—Cook County. 3. Intensive care units—Illinois—Chicago. 4. Intensive care units—Illinois—Chicago—Anecdotes. 5. Hospitals—Illinois—Chicago—Anecdotes. I. Title. II. Title: Cook County Intensive Care Unit.
    RA975.5.I56F73 2015
    362.17'4097731—dc23

                                2015018606

Cover design: Andrew Brozyna, AJB Design Inc.
Cover images: Shutterstock
Interior design: PerfecType, Nashville, TN
Interior layout: Nord Compo
Printed in the United States of America
5 4 3 2 1

CONTENTS

INTRODUCTION

"Life is short, and art long; the crisis fleeting;
experience perilous, and decision difficult."

—HIPPOCRATES

ONE COULD ARGUE that no profession has an older and richer literary tradition than medicine, and it is a tradition that has no geographical boundaries. Is it possible to say which country has produced the best writing about doctors and patients? Certainly Russia can make a claim. Tolstoy, Pasternak, Turgenev, and Dostoyevsky, among others, all wrote marvelously on the subject of medicine. But were they superior to the English—Conan Doyle, Emily Brontë, Thomas Hardy, George Orwell, et al.? And in any discussion of medicine in literature, the American literary canon bears consideration—Hemingway, Fitzgerald, Faulkner, Sontag. Those authors are just part of an impressively long American list, which carries on in the current era with people like Sherwin Nuland and Richard Seltzer.

My point is not to create some specious literary salon argument, but to illustrate the universality of the powerful emotions and personalities of the doctor/patient relationship. And as Norman Cousins observed in his 1982 classic *The Physician in Literature*, this is best illustrated in the anecdote:

the quotidian accounts from real life that occur any place where patients encounter doctors—hospitals, clinics, or the office. Cousins wrote:

> Writers are natural producers of anecdotes. This is what they are supposed to be. The anecdote is their stock in trade. We absorb these anecdotes and we learn from them. I now give a course in a medical school on the physician as perceived by the writer. Nothing is more interesting to me in that course than the willingness of students to take fictional anecdotes more seriously than they do examples from real life. Fortunately, by the end of the course, many of them come to recognize that even isolated incidents in human experiences can be repeated and are therefore significant.

Luckily for me when I undertook this book to recount my anecdotes, it was not necessary to have the literary skills of the aforementioned great authors. Over four decades, I was a medical student, medical resident in training, and then an intensive care and clinic physician at Cook County Hospital in Chicago. (Reflecting the values of our current age, the hospital has since been renamed John Stroger Hospital, after not a doctor but a politician.) Before that, my father worked at Cook County as an attending physician in the hospital's magnificent decade after World War II. So except for a brief hiatus in the turbulent 1960s, my family's experience covered most of the second half of the twentieth century and the first decade of the twenty-first—fifty years at one of America's premier urban hospitals.

Located on the city's Near West Side, Cook County Hospital has a storied history and is perhaps as famous as any hospital in the world. During my training, I received patients from six continents who traveled specifically to be treated at Cook County. (Regrettably, to the best of my knowledge no patient from Antarctica ever arrived for care at County.) The hospital was originally built to treat cholera patients in the middle of the nineteenth century, but the famous building on West Harrison Street, the facade of which still stands today, was built in 1916. One of the best historical accounts of the hospital is *The Old Lady of Harrison Street*, written by the eminent surgeon/author John Raffensperger, a medical student of my father, and my teacher when I was a medical student. Such was the tradition of care the hospital encouraged.

In terms of medical and nursing training, Cook County was one of the world's great teaching hospitals, especially in the 1940s and 1950s, when it was a nearly four-thousand-bed facility. There, doctors and nurses learned through clinical experience and seeing large numbers of patients, supplemented by reading books and listening to professors. University and community hospitals of the era were not so fortunate to have the same clinical volume. Because the best and brightest from all over the world were attracted to Cook County, it became an international center of medical instruction and research. A significant percentage of the American doctors and nurses who trained in the years after the war either spent time at County or learned from people who did. One of the world's first blood banks was opened there, and a number of surgical techniques were first pioneered there. The hospital developed a worldwide reputation in trauma, burn care, AIDS treatment, and intensive care, the last being the field that I elected to pursue for my career.

Just as important as their intellectual commitment, the doctors and nurses who were attracted to work there were fantastically dedicated and devoted to caring for patients. Most of them demonstrated a real love of humanity. The hospital was located in a poor neighborhood and was always available to everyone, regardless of ability to pay. It was one of the world's foremost charity hospitals for the poor and destitute. Many of these patients were brought in from the nearby neighborhood, but County also accepted great numbers of patients from other hospitals. These patients were generally transferred there because they were unable to pay for care. Nor was this an exclusively local phenomenon; poor patients not infrequently came from hospitals as far away as Mississippi and California.

The rich ethnic mixture of Chicago, then the country's second-largest city, made the hospital a veritable melting pot. In the mid-twentieth century, the wards were filled with immigrants from Eastern Europe, Italy, and

Ireland. Later the hospital became the primary health facility for thousands of African Americans who traveled by rail, bus, and car to Chicago as part of the great postwar migrations from the South. A sixteen-hour journey by a sick patient from Clarksdale or Greenville, Mississippi, to the hospital on Harrison Street in Chicago was not unusual. It was no exaggeration to say that Cook County was the hospital most trusted by the poor of the Mississippi Delta. (Although the hospital today is much smaller and has lost much of its intellectual luster, the phenomenon of poor patients coming from far away continues. Today, patients routinely come from Mexico, Central America, and South Asia; Italian and Polish translators are no longer as necessary as ones fluent in Spanish and Urdu.)

The plotlines in the County dramas are primarily about sickness and death, but there is an ongoing undercurrent of poverty, mental illness, alcohol, drugs, and crime in the stories. Certainly, no Hollywood writers' department ever had more elements of drama at its disposal. Even politics was a recurring subtext, as the hospital was a perennial political football for the Cook County Democratic Party, the most powerful political machine in the United States. Cronyism was ubiquitous. A telling example: years after mechanical elevators were installed at the hospital, elevator operators were still hired to run them manually. These low-level political operatives took long lunch breaks, received plenty of overtime pay, and got a paid day off on Election Day to work the precincts and make sure the Democratic vote was delivered. The elevator operators are now long gone, but patronage and union featherbedding persist even today.

Over the decades, Cook County has been fertile ground for fictional and nonfictional accounts by physicians and nurses. Like Al Capone and Michael Jordan, the name Cook County Hospital is inextricably linked to Chicago. With the possible exception of Massachusetts General in Boston and Bellevue in New York, no American hospital has been the backdrop for more books, articles, and movies. One of the more recent treatments of Cook County Hospital was the popular film *The Fugitive* (1993), directed by a Chicagoan. I was a technical adviser to the movie, and some aspects of what went into the movie are discussed herein. With the exception of a rollerblading orderly, it was a pretty realistic depiction of the hospital.

But my stories about the hospital are ultimately about the main characters: the doctors, nurses, and patients. This book is their story, and it covers more than a lifetime of personalities. Some of the more contemporary accounts are about patients unable to escape the poverty and violence of today's Chicago. One story dates back to my father's era of the early 1950s, when patients were brought to the hospital from the downtown train station during cross-country stops. And there is the strange tale of the long-ago hospital employee who worked in County's basement morgue for decades. The common thread in these very different stories is Cook County Hospital.

I have tried to avoid idealizing the patients, doctors, and nurses, as is sometimes the practice of books in this genre. I attempted to portray them as I saw them—as human beings, neither saints nor caricatures. Moreover, while most of the stories are from County Hospital, I have included some from other phases of my career in university hospitals. These include fascinating cases, illustrative anecdotes, historical observations, commentaries about American medicine, and some dark humor. Finally, I don't believe any book about medicine would be complete without providing the reader with some clinical information. Readers can come away feeling they have acquired a smidgen of medical knowledge. After all, medicine is best practiced when patient and physician understand each other by learning to speak the other's language. That is my hope with this book.

1

CLIMBING THE MOUNTAIN
OF MEDICAL SCHOOL
(AND FINDING IT IS JUST SNOW
AND ICE)

"I'll tell you what it's like to be No. 1. I compare it to climbing Mount Everest. It's very difficult. Lives are lost along the way. You struggle and you struggle and finally you get up there. And guess what there is once you get up there? Snow and ice."

—DAVID MERRICK

EVERY YEAR, THOUSANDS of undergraduates who have worked extremely hard during college apply to medical school. It is a highly selective process and only the top students are accepted. While admission to medical school is the first step to a successful career as a physician, once students begin their studies, they immediately find themselves at the bottom of the rigid medical hierarchy. As such, they are subject to the whole host of indignities that the medical education system can inflict. It is a tough road, even for those of the strongest character. One of the favorite pastimes of residents in training and attending physicians alike is to harass and intimidate those on the lowest rungs of the ladder, and of course that is medical students.

Surgeons are particularly fond of abusing students, especially in the operating room. It is extremely uncommon for the students to talk back, because there is just not much percentage in it. To illustrate why, there is a story of my classmate from the East Coast with a New York attitude. He was once assisting a general surgeon who was performing a gallbladder removal in the days before laparoscopic surgery rendered a bunch of surgical assistants unnecessary. A student's role in the operation is minor, since he or she doesn't have enough experience to do anything important. Generally, it means holding retractors during the operation to give the surgeon better vision of the operative field while he identifies the organs. In this case, my classmate had to hold a large retractor pulling back the liver that covered the gallbladder. This job requires holding and tugging for a long time. It is boring, and your arms get tired. But the medical student must not let go of that retractor while the surgeon is identifying and removing the gallbladder. And in most cases, the student has to remain absolutely quiet. *Speak only if spoken to.*

That day, the surgeon was taking a long time and the student was getting fatigued and frustrated. His surgical mask covered his face, but beads of sweat collected on his forehead. Suddenly, the frustration boiled over and he broke the unwritten rule. He asked the surgeon, "Well, how are we doing?"

The surgeon, and everyone else in the room, looked up. They were stunned. A medical student talking—and not just talking, but talking with impertinence.

The surgeon, taken aback momentarily, regained his composure and continued operating. But he was not about to let the transgression pass unnoticed.

He shot back to the student, "What do you mean *we*?"

That was a clear signal for the student to shut up immediately. Perhaps it was his New York attitude, but the student ignored the cue and fired back with thinly veiled sarcasm, "I like to think I'm as much a part of the health care team as anyone."

The surgeon, now fully engaged, had never encountered such braggadocio from a medical student, and he was prepared to enjoy the back-and-forth.

Now he taunted the student, "Part of the health care team? *You*? You must be kidding. You are nothing. We could get a monkey to do what you are doing. You are nothing."

The battle was on. No longer feeling subservient, the student challenged the surgeon. "Oh yeah? I'm nothing? I'll bet if I let go of this retractor, you would have trouble finishing the operation." He made a point not to let go of the retractor, though.

The operating room was silent. The surgeon then decided it was time to pull rank.

"I'll bet if you let go of that retractor, you'd have trouble graduating."

Point, set, match.

A couple of days later in the surgical locker room, the student told me he just lost his head in the heat of the moment. I asked him if the surgeon retaliated in any way. No, he said, the surgeon actually liked him and didn't hold it against him. The student survived the battle, graduated, and became a successful physician in Manhattan. But not every surgeon would have been so gracious.

———————

When I became an attending physician, it was not my style to harass or bully the medical students. I tried to help or encourage them whenever possible, figuring they were having enough trouble without grief from me. Once a student of mine, an especially earnest one, wanted to impress me.

So I gave him a difficult assignment: to draw blood from a hardened gang member. It was challenging because we needed to draw from an artery to test the oxygen level in the patient's blood, which a routine blood draw from a vein does not provide. It was a test of the student's skill.

The assignment was to draw blood at the patient's wrist, from the artery where you take your pulse. The artery is close to the bone, so if the needle misses the artery and hits the bone, it can be quite painful. And it's not a good idea to inflict unnecessary pain on a gang member, especially when you are a student. He went to draw the blood from the patient's artery, and it took fifteen long minutes. It must have been agony for the patient—and a different type of agony for the student. When the fifteen minutes were over, he had a sample from the patient, but unfortunately he had missed the artery and the blood sample was from the nearby vein, useless for the information we needed.

The student was disconsolate. Unaccustomed to failure in his academic career, he came to me knowing that he had failed and was worried that he had let me down. Besides that, we still didn't have the sample we needed. I reassured him, told him how difficult obtaining those samples was, and said we could still get an arterial sample. He told me there was no way the patient would let him try another needle stick.

"The last five minutes I was trying to draw it, he was staring me down. I don't think he will let anyone draw his blood now."

I said, "Don't worry, I will draw his blood. Come on, I'll take you with me."

"But what are you going to tell him?"

"Watch."

We went to the patient's room and, as predicted, he gave us a nasty glare. His right wrist was extremely sore from the unsuccessful blood draw.

"Man, what'chu guys want?" He suspected we were there to draw blood again.

"I have to take another sample, Andrew."

"Hey, he already drew my blood. What'chu need more blood for?"

The student was visibly nervous. He thought I was going to tell the patient he had made a mistake by getting an erroneous sample. It would be devastating to the student's already shaky confidence.

"Andrew, he got the sample from your right wrist. We saw the results. But we have to draw a sample from your left wrist to compare it with the one from your right. I know that one was painful, but don't worry, I'll draw this one. We have to see if the right and left blood are the same or different."

Of course, there is no difference between blood drawn from the left arm and the right arm. Same blood. But I gambled that Andrew didn't realize that. He gave me a suspicious look, considered the problem a minute and said, "OK, Doc. Go ahead."

I drew the blood from the artery of his left wrist quickly and painlessly.

"Thanks, Andrew."

"No problem, Doc."

Andrew nodded approvingly at me, and then at the student. The gang member was actually happy he could be cooperative. He was satisfied, the student was relieved, and I had the necessary sample. The student thanked me for rescuing him. He went on to become one of the country's top physicians in his field, far eclipsing me and my career. I wonder if he ever tells his students that story.

One of the final indignities of medical school is the interview for residency positions in the student's senior year. This is not always an unpleasant experience, because some hospitals want to attract the best students and thus treat them well during interviews. But in my case, coming as a student from Chicago and interviewing in the highly competitive atmosphere of New York hospitals, I was forced to run the gauntlet. Manhattan has some of the best hospitals in the United States, and it is a wonderful place to live when you're young and single, so I had decided to interview there for my residency. New York, New York—even for a medical student—if you can make it there . . .

It was right before Christmas. In Chicago, Mayor Daley—the first Mayor Daley—had just died. Chicago was grieving as I caught the early flight to La Guardia on a cold winter morning, greeted by a frigid wind whipping around the right angles of the downtown Manhattan skyscrapers. The morning of my first interview, I hailed a cab to St. Vincent's in Greenwich Village, a once-legendary hospital.

The legacy of St. Vincent's has faded, but in its day it was quite a grand place, one that recalled a different, more glorious era of medicine. Founded in 1849 with a mission to care for the poor and disenfranchised, it was world renowned for its care. The poet Edna St. Vincent Millay was named after the hospital. How many famous poets have been named after hospitals? Unfortunately, several years ago, after 163 years in business, the hospital closed unceremoniously, a victim of medicine's changing business environment.

But when I interviewed there in the 1970s, St. Vincent's was still a vibrant place. The intensive care unit was among the country's finest, and the hospital, which turned no one away, took care of the widest variety of patients: bohemians from the Village (the poet Dylan Thomas died there after a legendary bender); alcoholics from the Bowery; high-level professionals from the Financial District; and Chinese immigrants from Chinatown. Nobody knew it then, but St. Vincent's would soon become one of the major AIDS hospitals in the world, an ironic coincidence for a hospital that celebrated its strict Roman Catholic heritage.

The morning of my interview, I was sent to a basement cafeteria and told to wait there. I got a cup of coffee and sat down with a number of students from New York medical schools. It seemed they all were interviewing at the same hospitals and all knew each other. I was the nervous outsider, listening closely to the gossip about the pluses and minuses of the New York hospitals.

I was completely ignored until one of the students unexpectedly turned to me and asked in a thick Long Island accent, "So, wheah you from?"

"I'm from Chicago," I answered in my flat Midwestern tone.

"Oh, University of Chicaguh."

"No, actually, I'm from Northwestern."

This was my first taste of New York City provincialism. In those days, the common belief was that if you were from Chicago, you had to be from the University of Chicago. There were simply no other universities there. Saul Steinberg's famous *New Yorker* cover, "View of the World from Ninth Avenue," is not without some basis.

The student looked aghast, and proceeded to give me a geography lesson about exactly where my university was located. "Nawthwestun's not in Chicaguh, it's in Ohiuh."

One of his colleagues, looking to correct him, located Northwestern in the Great Northwest. "Nah, Nawthwestun's not in Ohiuh, it's in Warshingtun."

Thankfully, a resident with a slightly more refined Manhattan accent rescued me at that moment. "You can come with me, I'm going to give you a touah." A tour of the hospital, which I considered a pleasant gesture. How thoughtful.

It was still early, before 8 AM, and I figured my interview wouldn't be until at least 9. I relaxed a bit, opened the buttons on my sport jacket, and popped a stick of gum into my mouth, chewing unobtrusively while the resident led on. It was a mistake.

For the next ten minutes, the resident was sullen and rude. He didn't want to be there and answered no questions, but I found the hospital to be beautiful, immaculate and charming in its dotage. It was certainly cleaner than some of the new, Soviet-style hospitals at which I had interviewed. The hospital was festooned with Christmas decorations. A crucifix hung in every room, and there were reminders everywhere of the proud Catholic tradition of the Sisters of Charity, who had founded the hospital more than a century before. You don't see that much in hospitals anymore. It is a grand tradition all but gone from American medicine, never to return.

At the same time, I also sensed a real passion for patient care and quite a degree of medical sophistication and professionalism. Passion, sophistication, and professionalism with a tinge of rudeness—it's Manhattan. Even to a non-Catholic like me, the hospital was an extremely impressive place, and I saw why it had the reputation it did. I thought, "I would be proud to work here."

No chance of that happening.

About ten minutes into the tour, the dour resident brought me to a room and shoved me in with no warning. It was my interview. Unannounced.

The chief of medicine at St. Vincent's for many years was Dr. William Grace, the elderly scion of the Grace publishing family and one of the most brilliant cardiologists in the country. He was a pioneer in cardiac care and treatment for myocardial infarction—and, most notably, he founded the first mobile coronary care unit in America, basically a white-over-red Chevy van with monitoring and resuscitation equipment, capable of defibrillation. It could answer calls over a wide area of Lower Manhattan. While now routine, it was a revolutionary concept in the 1960s. It is a pity Dr. Grace is not better known today. He was a legend in his time, and he was one of the reasons I wanted to be at St. Vincent's.

And at that moment, he was sitting right in front of me.

To say the least, it was unanticipated—and intimidating. They say you don't want to meet your heroes because you'll be disappointed in them. In this case, it was the exact opposite. Flanked on each side by three nuns, he measured me up before I had time to swallow my gum and button my jacket. I certainly disappointed them.

It happened that Dr. Grace interviewed nearly every residency candidate personally. He died shortly after my interview, so I had the distinction of being one of the final candidates he ever interviewed; I think I also earned the distinction of having the shortest interview of all time.

He didn't ask me to sit down.

Since there was a chair in front of him presumably meant for residency candidate interviews, I took that as a bad sign.

He looked down at my résumé. "I see you are from Chicago."

"That's right, sir."

That was the high point. Everything went downhill from there. The nuns, who probably noticed I had been chewing gum, glared at me disapprovingly. They must have been wondering if there was a spare ruler around with which to rap my knuckles, or at the very least a couple of erasers for me to pound together after the interview.

Dr. Grace never looked up at me. He asked me one or two perfunctory questions and dismissed me summarily. Total interview time: four minutes.

I may have wanted St. Vincent's, but it was pretty obvious that St. Vincent's didn't want me.

There were still two other New York hospitals where I would interview that weekend. Columbia Presbyterian was different from St. Vincent's. It was, and is, one of the leading university medical centers in the country, prestigious doctors everywhere you turn. In truth, though, it was not as clean as St. Vincent's.

In my journey to and from Columbia Presbyterian, there was one incident I considered a potential omen. The hospital is on the north end of Manhattan, and my cab took the West Side Highway uptown. On the way there, I saw a nice, late-model car stalled on the side of the highway, no driver. I didn't think much of it. But this was New York in the 1970s. It was a different place from today, with a much rougher edge.

My "touah" and subsequent hospital interview took about two hours. I knew I was not at the top of their list; the university hospitals in New York got a tremendous number of applicants and had a preference for students from New York medical schools. After a short, unpromising interview, I was escorted to the hospital lobby, where I called a cab to head back to Midtown. The cab retraced the route on the West Side Highway. There, in the exact same spot, was the same late-model car I had seen abandoned a couple of hours before—now completely stripped, including the tires. Quite possibly a sign that New York wasn't for me.

My final interview was at Mount Sinai, located on the posh Upper East Side. To the south is one of the most affluent residential areas in the United States; to the north, Harlem is the site of some of the poorest neighborhoods in America. Mount Sinai is nearly as old as St. Vincent's, but is in no danger of closing. Its list of benefactors includes some of the country's wealthiest and most prestigious individuals, such as Wall Street power brokers Carl Icahn and Henry Kravis. This is reflected everywhere in the hospital.

Mount Sinai is beautiful, with long corridors and stunning hallways that feature its list of impressive donors. It was the first hospital designed by I. M. Pei. The clinical research at Mount Sinai has always been among the best in the country. It is the hospital where Crohn's disease and many other ailments were first described.

My chances of becoming a resident there were not good to begin with. The hospital had started its own medical school several years before and gave its students preference for residency. Besides that, I lacked the desired research background. But I had applied there and gotten an interview, so it was worth a shot.

Not for long.

I was given the obligatory brief "touah" of the hospital by another resident who was not interested in spending more than a moment with me. At least this one told me my interview would be coming up. He took me to a beautiful paneled room with a long walnut table and left me there. No one else was in the room, and I waited alone for about half an hour. Finally, an attending physician walked in, briefly introduced himself and sat at the other end of the table. I suspected the distance between us was not an accident.

He was smooth, with an air of enforced formality in his manner and more than a hint of imperiousness in his voice. For medical students from Chicago, Mount Sinai was not a place to be trifled with.

His first question was the same as at the other two hospitals: whether I was from Chicago. This was the one thing that had stood out in my folder in all three places. Unlike at the other Manhattan hospitals, this time I was able to elaborate on my answer with what I thought would be a point in my favor.

"Yes, my father worked very closely for years with Hans Popper."

Dr. Popper was a world-renowned Austrian liver specialist who fled the Nazis right before World War II and came to Chicago. My father worked with him at Cook County for many years before Popper left for New York, where he was named the chief pathologist at Mount Sinai. He was instrumental in founding the Mount Sinai School of Medicine and was appointed its first dean. Sometimes, that kind of connection helps. I thought it might impress my interviewer.

It didn't. In fact, it barely registered.

My father had offered to call Popper to help me secure a position there but I told him not to, because I wanted to earn it on my own. But when that got me no points, I had nothing to fall back on. I started wondering if I could get an earlier flight back to Chicago.

His final question was one I had not been asked before.

"How do you treat pulmonary edema?"

Occasionally in interviews, doctors will ask students clinical questions, as a way to ascertain how much the student really knows. Not every interviewer did it then, but today it is almost standard operating procedure. The practice never made sense to me, because every good student knows the basics of treating pulmonary edema (fluid in the lungs), but no student has the actual experience to give more than a superficial answer. It wasn't like physics, where a good answer to a theoretical question might let you pick out the really brilliant student who may have a special gift. Medicine doesn't work like that.

Others disagree, but I always felt that resorting to this type of question took away from what the interviewer really wanted to learn about the candidate—personality, character, interests, what type of resident he or she might become. Years later, when I interviewed candidates, I never once asked a clinical question. I felt it would be demeaning to the candidate, who, in truth, was applying to learn the exact thing you were asking him if he knew.

Back at Mount Sinai, I was quite capable of giving my interviewer an acceptable response, one that could pass an exam. I had treated enough patients with pulmonary edema to give him the superficial answer that you can get from reading a book, but I saw the question as a sign he was reinforcing the distance, literal and metaphorical, between us. Letting me know my place—and it wasn't Mount Sinai.

But in a sense, the question was liberating. The long day, quick tours, the stripped car, the paneled room, the walnut table, the dismissive attitude, and now this. I knew I didn't belong. And he knew I didn't belong. I gave him an answer I was pretty sure he had never heard before, and probably has not heard since.

"I guess if I knew how to treat pulmonary edema, I wouldn't be sitting here applying to learn how to treat it."

Like the medical student from New York in the Chicago operating room who held the retractor, I would have perhaps been better served holding my tongue. All of us say things we wish we had held back, and I have said more than my share. But this was not one of those times.

My answer was undoubtedly impertinent, bordering on disrespectful. But as Bob Dylan once said, "When you ain't got nothing, you got nothing to lose." And on that winter day on the Upper East Side of Manhattan, I had nothing and nothing to lose. I wasn't going to be accepted even if I were the world's expert on pulmonary edema.

He definitely wasn't expecting that answer. Caught off guard, his jaw dropped slightly and his preternatural calm was shattered for a brief moment. Then he regained the poise I'm sure he demonstrated in every meeting. He brusquely closed my file.

"Well, I think we are done." End of interview.

The medical student from Chicago left the bludgeonings of New York, head bloodied and slightly bowed. I never heard back from any of the three residency programs. Just another student indignity on the road to becoming a doctor.

2

MEDICATIONS CAN MAKE YOU (AND THE FISHES) SICK

"I firmly believe that if the whole *materia medica*,
as now used, could be sunk to the bottom of the sea,
it would be better for mankind and all the worse for the fishes."

—OLIVER WENDELL HOLMES SR.

HOLMES, THE NOTED nineteenth-century physician and writer, issued this critique of the medications of his day (then known as the *materia medica*) at an 1860 meeting of the Massachusetts Medical Society. Without question, the medicines prescribed in his era had a much greater chance of hurting patients than of helping them. That discouraging fact was probably true up until the middle of the twentieth century, when antibiotics were discovered. Today, pharmaceuticals are a multibillion-dollar industry, and physicians have access to a staggering array of medications, most of which are effective, many of which are lifesaving or at least symptom relieving. But one thing has not changed since Holmes's day: medications can still kill you, or at least make you sick. Even the best medication, in the wrong dose or prescribed at the wrong time, can be dangerous. It is an axiom physicians ignore at their peril—and, more important, the peril of the patient.

Just before my residency began, I was a student on the neurology service. By coincidence, a patient I happened to know was brought into neurology and I volunteered to be on the team taking care of him. He was a frail old man in his seventies, admitted for severe Parkinson's disease. His voice and the uncontrollable Parkinsonian tremor made him seem even older, and also made it difficult to evaluate whether he understood what was happening around him. It is sometimes hard to determine how attuned Parkinson's patients are to their surroundings. To most of the people on the service, he was just another old man. But at one time, decades before, he had been one of the most well-known people in America. No one on the team, from the attending to the residents to the interns to the nurses, knew who he was.

It's surprising how often that occurs. For the most part, doctors and nurses are young, and they may not know anything about a patient who was famous a long time ago. I saw it happen more than once when the old person was a formerly famous physician. This patient was not a physician, but for over forty years he had been a famous English professor at the university I attended, and that's why I volunteered to be on his care team. He was not just a famous professor but perhaps the university's *most* famous professor. He had written books, both scholarly and popular, and had been featured on television and radio panels and quiz shows (including the popular *$64,000 Question*, before it was tarnished by the 1950s quiz show scandals). He exchanged letters frequently with the world's leading intellectuals, including W. H. Auden and Ashley Montagu. His favorite correspondent was Groucho Marx, a closet intellectual, and judging by the frequency with which they wrote each other, Marx must have felt the same way about him.

The professor was once described in a national magazine as "an academic superman." He taught a renowned course, Introduction to Literature, three times a week in the university's largest lecture hall. It was so popular that the number of people who registered but never showed up to his course was greater than the number who attended any other course at the university. Over the span of forty years, thousands of students took his Introduction to Literature. I was one of those thousands, and my mother had taken his course in the very same lecture hall back in the 1940s.

It turned out the class I was in, only about five years earlier, was one of the last he taught before he retired. Unfortunately, he had deteriorated significantly since retirement. No doubt the onset of Parkinson's had much to with that. When I first examined him, he looked smaller and paler than I remembered, but of course my memory of him was watching him lecture to hundreds of students from a distant podium, where he seemed larger than life.

I was especially interested in how much he understood about what was going on around him. In assessing his mental status, I could tell he comprehended some things but not others. Of course he wouldn't remember me, but I mentioned to him that once upon a time I had been in his class, whereupon his masked face, a distinctive characteristic of Parkinson's disease, broke into a wan smile. Perhaps I reminded him of some long-ago student who approached him coming out of that lecture hall before World War II. Shades of *Goodbye, Mr. Chips*.

For obvious reasons, I spent more time with him than I did with any of my other patients. Gradually, I saw the tragedy: he understood his plight and was trapped inside a body he could no longer control. And he was aware, at least initially, that his mind—one of the best of his generation—was slowly ebbing away.

When I presented his case to the senior doctors, they seemed not to care that he was once a famous professor. It's not uncommon for senior doctors to pay little attention to students' presentations or notes. This is a mistake that bespeaks arrogance, since the student, despite his or her inexperience, often does the most thorough job of writing and recording the patient's condition. To them, it didn't matter what I said; he was just another elderly Parkinson's patient. And so they patronized him, which happens all the time to old people in the hospital.

Still, there were occasional signs of the old professor, like when a resident gave him a mental status examination. A standard part of the neurologic evaluation involves having the patient recite the presidents of the United States in reverse order to see how far back they can remember. So the resident asked the professor to name the presidents. He expected "Ford, Nixon, Johnson, Kennedy, Eisenhower, Truman . . ." but instead what he got was "Rockefeller, Ford, Agnew, Humphrey, Johnson, Nixon, Barkley . . ." The resident had no clue what the professor was reciting: the *vice presidents* of the United States in reverse order. At first, I couldn't tell whether the professor was doing it on purpose, but he kept reciting vice presidents all the way back to the Civil War: ". . . Wilson, Colfax, Johnson, Hamlin." He was demonstrating that he still had significant mental capacity. The clueless resident remained unimpressed.

After the evaluation, the neurologists decided to use a new drug to treat his Parkinson's disease. At first, the drug seemed to be working, as his movements became a little more fluid and his alertness picked up. But things rapidly deteriorated. He started to have hallucinations and became psychotic. He had never exhibited this type of behavior before, so to me the situation strongly suggested this was a side effect of the medication. Unfortunately, the doctors refused to believe that, even though his strange behavior was completely new and totally out of character. So they continued to give him the medicine.

This failure of doctors to believe that a new drug may actually be doing harm rather than good is a common problem. First of all, it can be hard to tell whether new symptoms are from the condition being treated or whether they are caused by the medication. Second, while good doctors keep an open mind, some simply refuse to believe a new symptom could be caused by the treatment they prescribed to the patient. (Likewise, some surgeons refuse to believe the surgery they perform can create new problems.) In this case, when I brought up the possibility that the uncharacteristic behavior was a medication side effect, it was summarily dismissed.

I came in to talk to the professor every day and watched him grow more psychotic as time went on. Further bolstering the impression was his appearance change. His hospital gown became disheveled, and the nurses didn't shave him every day, so the professor, once impeccably dressed, began to look like a homeless man. I thought back to his best lectures, which happened to be on the play he considered Shakespeare's finest, *King Lear*. The cruel irony: he began to resemble a mad Lear on the heath.

Yet, like Lear, he retained vestiges of sanity. While I talked with him, he would occasionally recite verses of poetry. Some verses were from poems he taught in his class. I remember the feeling he conveyed while reciting from memory A. E. Housman's "The Culprit": "The night my father got me / His mind was not on me . . ." No doubt in his drug-induced psychotic state he made other famous literary allusions that passed completely over my head.

His condition continued to deteriorate. It happened so quickly during his hospitalization that I was amazed the doctors didn't associate the mental deterioration of this brilliant man with the new medication. Sadly, they saw nothing but an elderly Parkinson's patient exhibiting psychotic behavior.

Years later, when I had more experience, I read about the drug he was taking. Psychosis did indeed turn out to be a side effect, but there was another aspect of the problem I never considered, and it had to do with why he may have reacted badly to the drug: he couldn't drink water.

When it comes to the simple act of drinking water, hospital patients are sometimes left to their own devices. Many older patients are unable to take in sufficient water on their own, so they often become dehydrated. The doctors may not want to insert an intravenous line for fear of infection, so it becomes a difficult balancing act keeping the patient hydrated. If the nurses and other caretakers on the ward are busy, and the family is not around, these patients suffer dehydration simply because there is no one to help them drink their water.

Because the Parkinson's disease caused severe tremors and difficulty swallowing, the professor could not drink without assistance. He did indeed get dehydrated, and his kidney function was reduced. For several days, the doctors counted on the new medicine to help him lift his glass and swallow, but it didn't happen. He wasn't strong enough.

Eventually the dehydration became severe enough that the doctors had to insert an intravenous line. But by this time, his kidneys weren't working efficiently. So the medication and the metabolic byproducts of the drug gradually built up to toxic levels in his body. This in turn made side effects like psychosis even more likely. It was a vicious cycle: the longer he got the medicine, the less able he was to drink, and the less able he was to drink, the more the medicines built up in his body, making him more psychotic. A general hospital rule is that *the longer it takes a patient's condition to improve, the more likely the doctors will write the patient off.* In this case, it was only a matter of time. And shortly thereafter, the doctors did lose interest in the professor and essentially wrote him off.

I saw him one last time, after I left the neurology service in early July, when the new residents were starting. Before I went to his room, I asked the new residents how the professor was doing.

"That psychotic old man with Parkinson's? He went really crazy last night. *Delusional.* Claimed he was hearing cannons and a war was going on outside. We're going to transfer him to long-term care."

Long-term care—over the long term, if you're lucky, you may get some care.

There was no point in pleading the professor's case with the new team. The "academic superman" was now just another crazy old man. I went in to see him. He may not have known who I was, but even in his psychotic state, he recognized a familiar face and asked where I'd been.

"What happened to you? I missed you."

"I'm sorry, sir. I'm working somewhere else now."

"That's too bad."

I asked him about the episode the night before. His voice quavered, "Terrible, just terrible. Cannons firing. Flares. It sounded like the storming of the Bastille. I was quite scared. A war going on outside." He was truly afraid of some imaginary invasion. The resident had correctly described the professor's delusion.

But before I walked out the door, something occurred to me. It was July 4. The night before, July 3, Chicago held a fireworks show on the lakefront outside the hospital. It was right above his window. He must have heard the explosions and seen the fireworks. In his psychosis he imagined cannons and revolution going on outside. The delusion was quite easily explained.

I shook his hand and thanked him for everything he had taught me. He nodded graciously. "Adieu, adieu, remember me."

From *Hamlet*.

I never saw him again, but I do remember.

We once had an elderly patient in the ICU with severe bedsores. She had decubitus ulcers, pressure sores that injure the skin and underlying tissue. The primary treatment is to keep them clean to prevent extension into deep tissues. Occasionally, however, even with good treatment, the ulcers may burrow deep into the muscle and even reach the bone. This particular patient had some of the worst sores I had ever seen.

Despite a superb job of care by the nurses, the sores continued to progress deeper. Meanwhile, the patient, who had been alert but immobile, lapsed into a coma and her kidneys began to fail. Her laboratory values began showing a strange pattern suggesting problems with her electrolytes. I called in the nephrologists to make sense of the situation, but they were at a loss to explain the patient's electrolyte problem and kidney failure.

When something unexplained happens to a patient in the hospital, always check his or her medications.

We check what the patients are taking by mouth and what they are getting intravenously. In this case, none of the prescribed medications seemed to be the cause of the problem. But what a patient absorbs through her skin is also medicine.

This woman's severe bedsores were being treated with Betadine, the dark liquid antiseptic surgeons often apply to the skin before they make an incision. Normally, only small amounts of Betadine are used, and when the skin is unbroken, little or none of the drug is absorbed internally. But in this patient's case, because the wounds were large and deep, the nurses had to use large amounts of Betadine to cleanse the open areas. This made it more likely the Betadine would be absorbed into the bloodstream. Betadine is a derivative of iodine. Could the patient be absorbing iodine from the wounds? Was the abnormal electrolyte problem and kidney failure a result of toxic levels of iodine in her blood?

Iodine levels are not routinely measured in laboratory; they require special testing. I asked the toxicologist team to immediately draw samples for iodine and send them to a special lab. Several days later, the levels came back hundreds of times higher than normal. No one had ever seen iodine levels remotely close to these. The toxicologists wrote up the case in a medical journal and gave our ICU team a mention:

> Absorption from povidone-iodine [Betadine] preparations after topical administration has been reported to be negligible, but an elderly woman had increased serum iodine levels with possible metabolic complications after povidone-iodine solution was applied to decubitus ulcers.

This was the first reported case of iodine toxicity from topical absorption of an antiseptic skin cleaner.

———

The concern about medications causing unanticipated problems is even more pertinent if you use a drug frivolously or unnecessarily. *The benefit of the drug must exceed the risk.* In the following case, I failed to observe this admonition, which led me to create a warning I dubbed Franklin's law.

The old woman had pulmonary edema, and when she arrived in the ICU, she was quite ill. Her lungs were full of fluid, she could barely breathe, and she was not getting enough oxygen. She responded well to the standard treatment, and eight hours later she was stable and doing well. Then, I made a fateful decision that stayed with me for the rest of my career.

One of the classic treatments for pulmonary edema used to be morphine. It relaxes the patient's breathing, lowers the blood pressure, and helps take the stress off the heart. Sir William Osler, regarded by many as the greatest physician of the twentieth century, called morphine "God's Own Medicine," and even Oliver Wendell Holmes Sr. made it an exception from his comments at the 1860 Massachusetts Medical Society meeting.

Morphine is not used that much anymore for pulmonary edema, because there are other, newer medicines that can be used. But I was curious to see if the woman's pulmonary edema would improve faster with a small dose of morphine. The truth was, she was doing well enough that she did not need the drug. I was administering it because I thought it would help her—but, also because I wanted to see how it would affect her breathing and her vital signs. I considered it a learning experience, because it would provide information that might be useful with future patients. But what I was doing was technically unethical, because even though it was an accepted drug for her condition, I was experimenting unnecessarily with her life.

Moreover, I knew I was experimenting. Things could go wrong—she might stop breathing or have a severe drop in blood pressure. However, the risk seemed very small, and I thought I could control the situation. The dose of morphine I administered to her was very small, enough to help the fluid in her lungs but extremely unlikely to cause her to stop breathing. However, just in case, I had the appropriate treatment ready. If her blood pressure dropped, I had all the necessary fluids and medicines to raise it immediately. And if all else failed I had the antidote to morphine ready at her bedside. With all these safeguards and giving such a low dose, what could possibly go wrong?

That's when I created Franklin's law.

I gave her the small dose of morphine; it did not stop her breathing and her vitals changed very little. She did not seem better or worse. I thought perhaps I should repeat the dose. Then suddenly, *my* heart almost stopped. Her lips began to swell, she started to itch, then wheeze and complain of shortness of breath. She reacted to the drug in a manner that I had never anticipated and that would not respond to the antidote: she had an allergic reaction to the morphine.

She might have died from the reaction, but fortunately it was mild. As I frantically prepared to treat her allergic reaction, it subsided on its own before I did anything. Twenty-five years later, I still remember the "*clong*" in my heart when that happened. Imagine if she had died of a treatable disease while she was improving, all because I deliberately gave her a medication she didn't need. Thankfully, because the dose of morphine was small and the reaction was short-lived, she recovered quickly. Within a half hour she was improving again. The next day she was ready to leave the ICU. I never told her what had happened.

Thus was born Franklin's law: *Never, ever, challenge nature and take chances with a patient's life by giving him or her unnecessary medications.*

In truth, Franklin's law is merely a variation on what the aforementioned Oliver Wendell Holmes described a century earlier:

> Some very silly people thought the old Doctor did not believe in medicine, because he gave less than certain poor half-taught creatures in the smaller neighboring towns, who took advantage of people's sickness to disgust and disturb them with all manner of ill-smelling and ill-behaving drugs. In truth, he hated to give anything noxious or loathsome . . . unless he was very sure it would do good—in which case, he never played with drugs, but gave good honest, efficient doses.

3

THE EMERGENCY ROOM AT NIGHT: RADIOACTIVE PATIENTS AND CHOCOLATE ALL OVER THE PLACE

"A safe night, I'm living in the forest of a dream
I know the night is not as it would seem
I must believe in something, so I'll make myself believe it
That this night will never go."

—LAURA BRANIGAN, "SELF CONTROL"

FOR MOST OF the twentieth century, emergency rooms in America were not staffed by physicians specifically trained to work there. It was not until the late 1970s that emergency medicine was established as its own specialty, with its own specifically trained doctors. But soon the specialty acquired a popular cachet. The 1990s television show *ER*, featuring young, energetic, sometimes frisky residents and nurses, became a big hit. Suddenly, emergency medicine turned into the field that medical students wanted to go into. ER doctors became the equivalent of medicine's rock stars. They were cool.

Television and the movies like to portray real life, but not *too much* real life. My children watched *ER* religiously. I, on the other hand, was never a big fan of hospital shows. (The only exception: one of the first doctor shows, an early 1950s effort I watched in reruns: *Medic*, starring Richard Boone, who later became Paladin in *Have Gun—Will Travel*. Richard Boone was cool.)

Occasionally while my kids were watching *ER* I would drift through the living room and offer some gratuitous comment like "That would never happen in a real ER" or "You know it's not really like that in the ER." I was met with withering glares and a putdown like "What do you know, dad? You're not even an ER doctor." At that point, it was time to leave the room. There was no point in arguing with television.

But I did know something about the ER. Although I was an intensive care physician by trade, early in my career, before emergency medicine became its own specialty, I worked in the emergency room quite often. When it did become its own specialty, I stayed on as a consultant and teacher to the ER residents and attendings, working with them on how to diagnose and treat serious intensive care problems.

Anyone who enjoys working in an urban emergency room will tell you that one of the allures of the place is that it attracts its share of unusual characters. This applies to both staff and patients—but especially patients.

Without question, the most unusual clientele come to the emergency room at night. In every ER where I ever worked, the nurses subscribed to the "full moon theory"—i.e., the really crazy people come out during the full moon. I don't buy it, and know of no credible data to support it, but go to any emergency room at night and mention that "it's a full moon" and you most likely will see staff nod in recognition at the urban medical myth.

One night while I was working in the ER—perhaps it was a full moon, perhaps not—a young man came in and was assigned to the junior residents. Several of them evaluated the patient for about an hour before they came to me, perplexed. They had no idea what to do. I told them to begin by making a medical presentation of the patient to me. The senior resident began the standard presentation.

"The patient is a twenty-three-year-old black male with a chief complaint that he is radioactive . . ."

I cut him off right there. That was the first time I'd ever heard that and a sign that a formal presentation was unnecessary. Better just to ask them what was going on with the patient. I asked the obvious question: "Wait a minute. He says he is radioactive?"

"Yeah."

"Does he have any exposure to radioactivity?"

"No. He's just a regular guy off the streets."

At that point, I was not looking for a strict medical assessment, so I asked, "Anything unusual about him? Is he crazy?" There seemed to be something of a conflict among the residents over the patient's sanity. One resident thought he was crazy, another didn't. Not enough information to go on.

"Is there anything positive on his physical exam?"

"No, he looks normal."

"So what did you guys do?"

"We drew labs on him. They are all normal. Chest X-ray is normal too."

"So what do you want to do with him?"

"I want to discharge him. Greg [the intern] wants to get a psych consult."

"What do you think I should do?"

The flummoxed resident said, "That's just it. We need your help. He refuses to see a psychiatry resident and he won't leave."

Sensing that I would be seeing the patient shortly, I asked him, "Why not?"

"He says he won't leave before he gets a test for radioactivity. He wants to see if he really is radioactive."

"A test for radioactivity?"

The resident explained, "He's already been to two hospitals and they just blew him off. They told him they don't have a test for radioactivity. I told him we don't have a test for radioactivity in the emergency room either. But he wouldn't leave. You have to see him."

So it was my turn. Working in the emergency room often demands creative solutions, and this was definitely a case that called for maximum creativity. What to do with a man who won't leave the hospital until he gets a test that proves he is not radioactive?

I went to the patient's room and observed him for a moment before introducing myself. He acted suspiciously, but not inordinately so, and otherwise appeared outwardly normal. He didn't seem crazy, but you never knew. I asked him a few medical questions and then he reiterated his desire to have a test for radioactivity. Two hospitals had already failed him. He was determined not to leave.

I left the room for a minute to talk to the residents. One of them asked, "What do you think?"

"I think it's pretty clear he is not going to leave until he gets a test for radioactivity."

"What are you going to do?"

"I'm going to give him a test for radioactivity. Wait here."

Now the residents looked at me like I was the one who was crazy. There was no such thing as a routine test for radioactivity.

I walked back into the room and took the pager off my belt. In those days, the devices were simple beepers that sounded a tone if you were paged. But if you pressed the answering button on the beeper to test it, it made a static hiss like an open police microphone—or a Geiger counter. Holding down the button would create a continuous static hiss until the button was released. I approached the patient and told him to stand facing the wall. I made up some medical nonsense about a "level A radioactivity test" and pressed that button on my beeper. I ran the beeper up and down his back and he heard the static noise. Then I asked him to turn around and I ran the beeper down the front of his body. If nothing else, it certainly looked and sounded like a test for radioactivity. When I was done, I released the beeper, looked at him and said, "Nope. Nothing. You're all clean. No sign of radioactivity."

The young man was convinced and heaved a huge sigh of relief. Then he smiled at me and thanked me profusely. In thirty years, I never met a more thankful patient. He walked out of the room and his gratitude extended to everyone, doctors, nurses, orderlies. He shook everyone's hand and left even before we could finish the paperwork. A load had been lifted from his shoulders.

The residents were amazed. One of them asked, "How did you do that?"

In response, I took my beeper and "tested" the resident for radioactivity the same way. "That's the 'level A radioactivity test.' See, looks like you're clean, too."

Everyone laughed, but then I explained that the patient told me he had been to a clinic recently with a stomach complaint resembling an ulcer. He told me the clinic had him swallow something and afterward they took X-rays. It must have been a barium swallow; before endoscopes were common, this was how doctors obtained images of the stomach. Barium, while inert, was radiopaque, meaning it would show up on an X-ray. When the patient complained that he was radioactive, he was most likely concerned that the barium had not passed out of his body. I didn't think it would do any good to show him his chest X-ray or explain to him about barium swallows, so I had to give him the quick portable beeper radioactivity test.

The staff congratulated me on my quick thinking and a job well done. Everyone was happy until I said, "There's one thing that bothers me."

One of the residents who had learned a new radioactivity test asked, "What?"

I said, "What happens if he comes to another hospital ER, demands a quick test for radioactivity, and the doctors tell him there is no such thing?"

"So what?"

"The first thing he will say to them is 'The doctors at County have one and they gave it to me.' What do you suppose their doctors will think? How are we going to look when he says that?"

———————

Quick thinking saved the day in the ER in that case, but not long after that, I turned out to be too smart for my own good. That's the way medicine is. Humbling. You do something good, make a great diagnosis or perform a difficult surgery, and you think you can do nothing wrong. You're bulletproof. It's a dangerous feeling, because something will come along, probably sooner rather than later, and knock you off your perch. You will make an error or do something really stupid. That's why it is important to maintain an even keel—never too high or too low. Equanimity—it means imperturbability, and Sir William Osler considered it the most important quality of a good physician. Move past your successes quickly. There will be time to savor them later in life. Of course, the even keel also works the other way. If you wind up making an error or doing something wrong, you have to learn from it and forget it quickly. If you dwell on it, you can become paralyzed with indecision. The cat who got burned on a hot stove will never sit on a hot stove again. But neither will it sit on a cold one.

The case that humbled me after my radioactivity triumph happened on another night in the emergency room. It began at about 2 AM, when I got a call from another hospital to accept a transfer. The patient was a diabetic man who had tried to commit suicide by injecting himself with an overdose of insulin. The insulin would drive the man's blood sugar very low and fatally damage his brain. (An insulin overdose was the centerpiece of the notorious 1982 trial of Claus von Bülow, who was charged with the attempted murder of his wife, Sunny.) The overdose is easily treatable with administration of glucose, but the drop in blood sugar can recur hours later, after the body metabolizes the glucose.

Since the other hospital could not tell us exactly how much insulin the man took, it was uncertain how long glucose would have to be administered, and how long the man would have to be observed before the insulin effects wore off. His blood sugar could drop again at any time.

If he'd had insurance, the other hospital would never have transferred him. I was uncomfortable having a patient like that put in a transfer ambulance in the middle of the night; too many things could go wrong. But the doctors at the other hospital assured me of several things: he was stable, after their treatment his blood glucose was measured as normal, and they were administering concentrated glucose intravenously while he was in transport. It was a fairly short trip by ambulance from that hospital to County, less than half an hour. So I agreed reluctantly, even though no one knew how long the insulin in his body would keep acting to lower his blood sugar.

When he got to County, I made him the highest priority and evaluated him myself. It was about 3 AM. He was indeed stable, alert and able to talk to me, with an intravenous of concentrated glucose running in his arm. He could not remember how much insulin he had taken; he had passed out instantly. I had his blood sugar tested immediately and it was normal. Perhaps I should have been apprehensive, since with all that glucose running in his veins, his blood sugar should have been higher than normal. But I dropped my guard ever so slightly.

I noticed his face was bruised, he had a fresh scalp laceration, and there was evidence of trauma to his upper torso. He didn't remember how he got the trauma, but apparently before he was discovered the insulin overdose caused a hypoglycemic (low blood sugar) seizure. When he fell, he incurred the trauma. At that point, I made a bad mistake: arrogance. I decided to send him to radiology for X-rays of the trauma.

The inviolable rule of any emergency room, and any intensive care unit, is that unless you are absolutely certain of a patient's stability, you do not let him out of your sight or the sight of someone who knows how to manage an emergency. Make sure he is stable before sending him anywhere he can't be treated immediately. Especially at night.

It was 3:30 AM. This patient seemed stable, he had survived an inter-hospital transfer, he was talking to me, and he had lots of glucose running in his veins. I felt comfortable that I could send him down to radiology.

Since it was the middle of the night, there was a skeleton shift on, and there would be only a transporter—no nurse or doctor—to accompany him to X-ray. But the whole process should take no longer than an hour. He would probably be OK for that interval.

Now, in the back of my mind, I knew I could be violating the "unstable transfer" rule—at his peril. And I knew things could go wrong and it might take longer to get the X-rays. But I was in "I can do nothing wrong" mode and believed that everything would be fine. Still, I wasn't completely reckless and I hedged my bets. I gave him several extra injections of glucose. I started a new concentrated intravenous solution, guaranteed to run all the time he was in radiology.

And then the final touch. Before I sent him to radiology, I stopped in the cafeteria and went to the candy vending machine. I bought two Mars bars, partially unwrapped them, and gave them to the patient.

"Mike, while you are in X-ray, if you feel lightheaded or like your blood sugar is getting low, here are some candy bars. Just pop them in your mouth. Understand?'

"Sure, Doc, thanks." He smiled a reassuring smile. As a diabetic, he knew the drill if his blood sugar dropped. What could go wrong?

Looking back, I know I should have dispensed with the X-rays and admitted him to the hospital right then. It was 3:45 AM.

The transporters took him off to X-ray and I began working on other patients. I lost track of him. He was not back in the emergency room at 4:30 AM. Or at 5:30 AM. Or at 6:30 AM. I knew nothing really bad could have happened, because my cardiac arrest beeper had not gone off. The shift would end at 7 AM and I just figured the X-rays took longer than expected, a routine annoyance. At 7 AM I planned on going down to radiology and bringing him back.

Everything was quiet in the emergency room at 6:55 AM, when the new shift of doctors and nurses began filing in for "sign over," the transfer of care of all the remaining patients in the ER. Suddenly, all hell broke loose. The nurses wheeled in a patient having a grand mal seizure. I was in charge for another five minutes, so I began the resuscitation. The patient had a hospital gown and a hospital ID bracelet, so clearly he was not a new arrival from an ambulance.

As I performed resuscitation, I was assisted by the new crew of doctors and nurses. The last shift had signed off. Someone asked where the patient was from and the charge nurse said, "He was in radiology getting X-rays when he started seizing. We brought him back up right away."

Another "*clong*" to my heart—I knew immediately who it was. During resuscitation, you tend not to look too closely at a patient's face, because there are so many other things to do. But once I heard that, one look at his face provided confirmation. It was the patient with the insulin overdose I had last seen three hours ago. *You should not break the unstable transfer rule.*

Then the final indignity.

While we were doing resuscitation, one of the younger doctors said, "He must have lost control of his bowels in radiology. There's feces all over him." Everyone looked at his right side and recoiled slightly.

I looked at them and said, "It's not feces."

A nurse said, "It looks like feces. If it's not what is it?"

I said, "It's chocolate. Trust me. I know it's chocolate."

They looked at me strangely, but I knew what had happened. When the patient was in radiology, right before he had the seizure, he had taken the partially wrapped chocolate, unwrapped it, and tried to pop it in his mouth. Before he could do so, his blood sugar dropped, he began seizing, and the seizure caused him to crush the chocolate clutched in his hand. I was witnessing the consequences of my bad decision to let him out of my sight.

Everyone in the room looked at me strangely. Of course, not a single person believed it was chocolate, but it didn't matter. Fortunately he was resuscitated and cleaned off thoroughly. (The disbelieving staff cleaned off thoroughly as well.)

He was admitted STAT to the intensive care unit. He regained consciousness but continued to have intermittent hypoglycemic seizures for three days. He must have taken hundreds of units of insulin, a huge amount, in his suicide attempt. He was eventually discharged in good condition and I never heard about him again.

Mars bars used to be my favorite chocolate bar. But since that ER shift, I have never eaten one. In fact, now, even years later, every time I see one, I think, *"Never transfer a patient out of your sight if you are not positive he or she is stable."*

4

DEAD MEN DON'T TELL TALES, BUT SOMETIMES THEY GET X-RAYS AND ECGS

"It's not that I'm afraid to die,
I just don't want to be there when it happens."

—WOODY ALLEN

MOST PATIENTS WHO die in the hospital are either sick from a chronic disease or acutely and severely ill. When a patient dies it is usually expected, or at least not a surprise. But occasionally a death happens unexpectedly and it is a shock to the whole staff. The classical scenario is that it tends to happen late at night; the patient dies in his room after the night shift nurse looks in on him for the last time. When the morning shift comes on at 7 AM, the nurses start reviewing the reports on all the patients before seeing them. Meanwhile, the patient in 2355 is dead and no one realizes it. Any tests scheduled the night before have not been canceled and are about to be carried out.

It just so happened that in this case, the patient in 2355 who had died the night before was scheduled for a morning chest X-ray. Some X-rays are ordered as in-room X-rays that can be done at bedside by a technician using a portable machine. But on this occasion, the patient was scheduled for a two-view X-ray, which meant bringing him down on a gurney to the radiology department and having him sit upright to obtain two views, front and back.

Sure enough, at 7:30 AM, before any day-shift nurse had seen the patient, a transporter came in to wheel the patient to the radiology department. Apparently the transporter, who was occasionally known to take the morning to sober up after a late evening, didn't notice that the patient did not move or offer any resistance when he was placed on the wheeled stretcher. Or that underneath the blankets, he was cold to the touch. So the bleary-eyed transporter put the patient on the gurney and took him down to X-ray.

The radiologist, who was probably at the top of his class in medical school, happened to notice the patient wasn't moving. He examined the patient, and observed he was stiff. And cold. Radiologists are not used to making diagnoses—often that's why they went into radiology—but this one, unafraid of stepping outside his specialty, made a quick and accurate diagnosis: *the patient was dead.* For the radiologist, this was no small accomplishment; he hadn't seen a dead patient since his residency. He then went further and took the initiative to make an executive decision by canceling the X-ray. Unfortunately, he wasn't sure exactly who to inform of his diagnosis, so he called the senior physician he knew in the hospital—me.

I came down to radiology and immediately confirmed the diagnosis: "He's dead all right." I congratulated him on his diagnostic acumen and saw him swell with pride.

As I made arrangements to get the body to the morgue, the radiologist approached me. Considering what had just happened, he was remarkably nonchalant. I think he was feeling a little full of himself, being the one who figured out the patient was dead, so he let his sense of humor kick in. He didn't get many opportunities like this, and he wasn't about to let it pass.

"Dr. Franklin, the next time you want to get an X-ray on a stiff, do me a favor, order a portable X-ray. I don't do two-views on dead guys."

Radiologist humor. Of course, our joke about radiologists was that their official flower was the "hedge."

Another time, a terminally ill patient was admitted to the open ward. He had an intravenous line that was placed in the emergency room and oxygen by mask, but he was dying. Death was imminent and expected. He had a do-not-resuscitate order in his chart so that when his heart stopped no attempt would be made to revive him. Shortly after being admitted, he died. The nurse called me over to pronounce him dead, which I did, and she was about to take his intravenous line out and remove his oxygen when she was called away urgently to another patient.

So there was this dead man, lying in bed on the open ward with an oxygen mask and an intravenous line running, when the electrocardiogram (ECG) technician came over to do an ECG. He hooked up the ECG leads, and since the patient was still warm, the tech didn't think much of the fact that he wasn't moving. I was with some students who were about to tell the technician that the patient had expired, but I sensed my opportunity and held the students back.

"Just let the tech do the ECG."

They looked at me strangely. Why would I do that?

Of course the ECG was a flat line; dead people don't have any cardiac electrical activity. But the tech apparently didn't notice that—or, more likely, he didn't care. He left the ECG readout on the desk next to the patient and went off to do his next one.

I seized the moment. At the other end of the ward, oblivious to all this, was one of our most pompous, preening residents. I told the students before approaching the resident, "Let's see what happens."

I walked over to the resident, and, in my most earnest voice said, "Mark, that patient in the first bed, the one with the oxygen, looks a little pale. I think he may be having a myocardial infarction"—a heart attack. "Could you check out his ECG on the desk? If he's having an MI, we're going to have to bring him down to the ICU."

The resident didn't like me but was impressed that I would accord him such responsibility. I had given him authority. He walked over rather quickly, and did exactly what I hoped he would do.

Part 1. Instead of examining the dead patient, he went straight for the ECG. He looked at the flatline ECG.

Part 2. Again, he responded predictably: he didn't believe the ECG. Since dead people rarely get ECGs, the most common cause of a "flatline" is a loose recording lead on an arm or leg, or alternatively, a faulty machine, which is what the resident assumed.

Part 3. He called the ECG tech back and berated him.

"What's wrong with you? This ECG is flat. Is your machine working?"

The ECG tech was cowed, and I felt a little sorry for him. He was genuinely puzzled and assured the resident he had done two more ECGs since then, and had no problem with his machine. This just infuriated the resident.

Part 4. "Well, then do another ECG on that patient!"

By now my students were enjoying the show. Unwittingly, the pompous resident had just ordered an ECG on a dead person. While the ECG tech was hooking the patient up (the tech, not overly bright, had still not figured out the patient was dead), my students started snickering. Until then, the resident had reacted predictably. At this point, I had no idea what would happen next.

The resident stood over the tech while he did the ECG, and again he saw a flatline. This time he believed there was indeed no heartbeat. But he didn't realize that the patient had been dead for ten minutes, and he didn't know there was a do-not-resuscitate order. He simply assumed the patient had just had a cardiac arrest.

Part Five. He called a "code"—an emergency resuscitation procedure.

"SOMEONE CALL THE ARREST TEAM. THIS PERSON IS HAVING A CARDIAC ARREST!"

At this point, my students were laughing. The resident was calling for resuscitation on a dead patient. Then I had to step in.

"Mike, maybe you should listen to his lungs, see if he's breathing."

Part 6. He looked at me quizzically, took his stethoscope, and put it to the patient's chest. Naturally, he heard nothing, and then he realized the patient was dead and had been dead for several minutes. It took him about five seconds to put together what had happened.

He just sneered and uttered an obscenity under his breath directed at me.

I didn't hear the imprecation because my students, who never got much of a chance to make fun of a resident, were by now laughing out loud.

I actually got the idea for that little trick I had played on the pompous resident from something that had happened to me years before. When I was a young resident, one of our responsibilities was to "work up" preoperative patients who were scheduled for elective surgery. At that time, the surgeons required that all patients coming into the hospital for surgery, even for simple procedures, had to have a history and physical examination before their operations. This workup was a screening for any medical problems that might arise during surgery.

A generation before, the surgeons did their own preoperative examinations for routine operations. Eventually, most surgeons abandoned routine preoperative workups and, unfortunately, many of them abandoned routine postoperative care as well. Surgeons today (except for the good ones) are often only interested in what happens in the operating room. Before and after the operation, the patient is someone else's responsibility. So it fell to us lowly internists to do the medical evaluations before the patients went to surgery (just as it often fell to us to take care of them after surgery).

One night early in the evening shift, in my role as medical screener, I was examining an elderly man who was being admitted for a minor procedure: removal of a hemorrhoid. The patient was healthy, and the whole thing was quite routine. Suddenly, my pager went off for a cardiac arrest somewhere else in the hospital. Back when the day shift ended, the resident who was in charge of the resuscitation team had handed off the "code beeper" to me, and it was my responsibility to answer any cardiac arrest calls that evening. I quickly excused myself from my patient, told him I would return soon, and went to the resuscitation at the other end of the hospital.

When I arrived at the room of the patient who had arrested, the resuscitation was already underway. I was the senior medical officer, so it was my job to coordinate the effort. The patient, whom I knew nothing about, was hooked up to a portable ECG machine that had just been wheeled into the room. In those days, every room did not have cardiac monitors, and I was forced to make decisions as to what drugs to use and when to use the defibrillator based on the information from the continuous ECG readings from the portable machine.

Things did not go well. For nearly half an hour, despite frantic chest compression, a battery of drugs, and intubation, we had no success at restoring the patient's heart activity. All the ECG ever showed was a flatline. In medical parlance, it was called asystole: no heartbeat.

We worked for another ten minutes on the patient. When we had gone nearly forty minutes with a flatline ECG and no evidence of a heartbeat, it was my decision as the senior physician to "call the code": i.e., end the resuscitation effort and declare the patient dead.

At that point, because I always wanted to be sure, I took one last look at the ECG. It was still flatline, so I asked someone to feel for a pulse. There was none, so I "called the code" and ended the resuscitation. Calling the code was a routine I knew well.

"The clock says 5:57 PM, so that's the official time of death. I want to thank everyone. You did a great job. I'm just sorry we could not save the patient."

The nurses set about removing the patient's intravenous lines and preparing the body. The patient's resident thanked me, saying he would write a long note in the chart explaining the circumstances and would notify the family. There was nothing more for me to do but sign the resuscitation sheet, attesting to the time and details of the death.

Once that was done, I wanted to get some dinner, but first I had to head back down and finish the preoperative evaluation of my surgical patient. Nothing difficult, and wouldn't take more than a couple of minutes. If I was lucky, I could finish before the cafeteria closed. I completed the history and physical exam and drew his blood (in these days we had to draw blood from patients ourselves on off-hours).

The last thing to do before sending him to the surgical ward was to get an ECG. Unfortunately, it was after hours and there was no ECG tech around. The surgeons would not accept him without a preoperative ECG, which I would have to obtain and interpret. Without a tech, I was forced to do the ECG myself. Today, a physician doing an ECG, let alone a blood draw, is unheard of. Another example of how medicine has increased its specialty roles.

Unfortunately, there was no ECG machine in the preop area. There were also no nurses to tell me where I could find an ECG machine. I knew of only one ECG machine available: the one we had used minutes before in the cardiac arrest. So I trudged back over to the ward on the other side of the hospital, and sitting there was the ECG machine we had used. I told the nurses I had to take it over to the preop area. I would just be borrowing it and would return it after dinner.

I wheeled the machine all the way back down to the preop area and told my patient we would be finished as soon as we obtained an ECG. I instructed him to lie on the examining table, and remove his shirt and trousers so I could affix the leads to him and record the ECG. (Coincidentally, my father was one of the people who invented the old suctions that attached to a patient's chest to obtain the readings for the ECG. That old machine still used them, so for me, taking the ECG was a reminder of my heritage.) Once I had the machine attached I began recording the ECG. The readout of the patient in front of me, smiling and talking, showed no cardiac activity.

Nothing. Flatline. Asystole.

That clearly could not be the case, since the patient was obviously alive and comfortably resting on the examining table. After making sure the leads were placed appropriately, I repeated the ECG. Absolutely no cardiac activity.

Nothing. Asystole. Flatline.

The explanation was obviously that the ECG machine was faulty. Finally, a nurse came by and told me where I could get another machine, and I repeated the ECG. With the new machine, his ECG was normal and I sent the preop patient up to the surgical ward for his operation.

At that point, something occurred to me. The faulty ECG machine was the same one I had used minutes before to make decisions on resuscitation in a patient in cardiac arrest. It showed a flatline then, and the flatline it showed now was obviously a mistake. Was it in error an hour earlier when I had declared the patient dead? Could the first patient have been alive? Although there were other indications that the patient was truly dead, that broken ECG machine has always bothered me. Maybe the flatline on the first patient was false.

I will never know for sure. I passed on dinner that night. I suddenly had no appetite.

———

Sometimes dead men tell no tales because death comes quickly and unexpectedly right in front of your eyes.

One evening an unfortunate construction worker was brought in with an unusual but not unheard-of problem. He had been working at a construction site not far from the hospital when a piece of steel pipe fell several stories and pierced his skull. He was alive but in a deep coma when he was admitted. He was taken directly to the operating room with a foot of pipe protruding from the top of his head and another foot protruding behind his jaw.

Neither the junior neurosurgeon nor his staff had ever seen anything like this before. The patient was obviously dying in front of them and they had no idea what to do about the pipe. This happened nearly forty years ago so, of course, there was no Internet to search. The neurosurgeon was forced to make a quick decision. He decided to remove the pipe from the patient's skull.

Today, neurosurgeons with experience believe the best thing to do is to cut off as much of the ends of the pipe sticking out of the body as possible, cauterize the area, then gradually inch the pipe out to minimize the pressure shifts in the brain. Simply to pull the pipe out of the skull in one thrust, no matter how logical it seems, is definitely the wrong thing to do.

Unfortunately, the team didn't know this. Everyone was quietly stunned by the scene confronting them. The neurosurgeon looked around the room and said, "Anyone know what we should do here?'

Silence.

The neurosurgeon then said, "Well, if no one has a better idea, I think we'll go ahead and just pull it out."

The patient was quickly anesthetized and then the surgeon and one of the other residents just took the end of the pipe protruding from the top of the skull and pulled it out.

In less than thirty seconds, before the surgeons even had time to put the pipe on a surgical specimen table, the patient was dead. The patient's brain herniated through the bottom of the skull. The neurosurgeon looked up at the whole team, speechless for a moment.

Then he took off his mask and gloves and said, as matter-of-factly as possible, "Well, that wasn't the right thing to do."

No one said a word, and everyone slowly filed out of the operating room.

5

THE TOUGHEST MAN
IN THE HOSPITAL BECOMES
THE MOST PITIABLE

"Without hesitation Dove chose the nowhere road. For that was the only place, in his heart of hearts, that he really wanted to go."

—NELSON ALGREN

AS FAR AS "handles" on the street went, the toughest characters were all invariably known by their full first names. In the world of the street gang, appellations evolved in the opposite direction from how they developed back in grade school: nicknames did not inspire fear, so Andy became Andrew and Rick went by Richard. In the 'hood, it was your full name that conferred gravitas and meant you were a serious dude on the street.

About 1982, one really serious guy happened to become my patient. He was logged into the hospital as Jeff, but his street name was, of course, Jeffrey. The first time he came to the hospital he was about twenty-three, with a huge Afro, piercing blue eyes, and a fierce visage projecting an air of menace to all who came near him. *Don't make eye contact and don't come too close.* Think Samuel L. Jackson in *Pulp Fiction*, but meaner—much meaner.

To Jeffrey, the hospital was merely an extension of the street. No matter if you were a doctor, a nurse, or another patient, his scowl, if directed at you, left no doubt that to mess with him was to do so at your own peril. Unless one had medical business with him—to draw his blood, take his vitals, or see him on rounds—you were best off avoiding him.

Jeffrey was a street gang member and a heroin addict, and nakedly unapologetic on both counts. He was in the hospital for abscesses on his legs from needle use. His skin had sloughed from drug injections, and he required intravenous antibiotics and evaluation for skin grafting.

Occasionally, he would receive visitors in the hospital. They were also a menacing bunch, most likely his associates in the street gang. There was no question he was the alpha, and perhaps they came to deliver drugs to him (a frequent transaction in the hospital), or maybe they were just there to confer on business affairs sinister. While Jeffrey waited for his skin grafts, I would see him every day on rounds as his attending physician. Like everyone else, I adhered to the unstated protocol of the street: no eye contact. But part of my job as a physician was to understand the patient, and I was used to treating drug addicts. I gradually earned a modicum of Jeffrey's trust and he granted me the privilege of talking with him. Nevertheless, I still hesitated to make eye contact. The rules of the street could be enforced at any time.

In the hospital, no less than out of it, dealing with gang members and heroin addicts is invariably a precarious proposition. Physicians are authority figures, and gang members, by their very nature, distrust authority figures. It's not on the level of their interactions with the police, but it's a close second.

One of the best illustrations of this is the doctor's coat. A subtle difference between working at a county hospital and a university or suburban hospital (I have done both) is the doctor's coat. It is a uniform of sorts, meant to inspire trust. At university and suburban hospitals it generally fulfills that function, at least among most patients and staff. Wearing the coat gives you respect; people who don't know you smile and say hello. But at the county hospital the physician's coat sometimes has the opposite effect, especially with patients like Jeffrey. Official uniforms of any type are regarded with suspicion. As a symbol of authority, the coat represents a barrier. For this reason, sometimes I would go without my coat on the wards. Not wearing a coat would be unthinkable in the university hospital.

The other part of that equation was a lesson I learned the hard way: that heroin addicts can rarely be trusted. They are clever and manipulative. Early in my career, in my naïveté, I would fall for some cockamamie sob story and loan some drug-addicted patient five dollars. He would invariably promise to pay me back. Of course, not a single one ever did, and this learning experience cost me about fifty dollars before I adopted a new personal policy: no more loaning money to drug addicts, no matter how dire their story. Most of my colleagues, who were less trusting to begin with, never fell victim to those scams. Live and learn.

Some of these addicts could take their ruses to incredible limits. I once saw a young man in the emergency room fake abdominal pain. Since his veins had been destroyed by the constant injection of drugs, the doctors had to insert an intravenous line in his jugular vein, a large vessel in his neck—a minor surgical procedure. However, once the open vein was established, the patient simply walked out of the hospital with the intravenous line still in his neck when no one was looking. The abdominal pain turned out to be nothing more than a ploy to have the doctors establish a useable vein into which he could inject street drugs.

In the same vein, excuse the pun, another addict once told me there was an enterprising and talented amateur in his neighborhood. This guy could use a syringe to find a vein in addicts when even the doctors failed. His basic charge was ten dollars per customer. Word was he did a thriving local business in the niche industry of finding usable veins. I always wondered if perhaps he had become the beneficiary of some of my loan money.

One afternoon in the last days of Jeffrey's hospital stay, I came by and asked if we could talk. He eyed me up and down suspiciously but then nodded his assent and pointed to a nearby chair, signifying that I should pull it up next to his bed. He tended to communicate primarily with gestures. When he did speak it was usually in short, terse sentences.

"What'chu want, man?"

"Nothing, just want to find out how you are doing. If you need anything."

"I'm OK. I could use some more pain medicine."

Standard request from addicts. "Sure, I'll take care of it."

Whether he needed more pain medicine or not, it was worth the price of prescribing him more to gain his trust. In that case, the doctor/patient manipulation was mutual.

"Jeffrey, how much heroin do you use?"

I knew he might not answer that question, but if he did, his answer would be in a dollar amount. I wanted to get a rough idea of the extent of his habit. Of course, the correlation between what he said and what he used was probably imprecise. Almost all heroin users exaggerate the actual amount they use. To my mild surprise, he was not reluctant to answer; I considered this a display of trust.

"'Bout $100 a day."

Even if it was half as much, this was a significant habit in those days. This also told me that, although he may have been a fairly high-ranking and feared street gang member, his extensive drug use would eventually be an impediment to his rise in the organization. A top capo could not function with that kind of addiction.

"Where do you get that kind of money?" I was familiar with most of the answers to that question, but I was curious to see what he would say. Young male heroin users had a wide range of ways, violent and nonviolent, to support their habit. Older men who were not as physically agile were more apt to commit some sort of fraud. Writing bad checks was especially common. Meanwhile all but the oldest female addicts gravitated toward shoplifting or prostitution.

Jeffrey was quite direct. "Different things: selling, boosting." He smiled and continued, "Sometimes I get it from guys like you."

I didn't know what he meant by that remark and I was slightly taken aback.

"Guys like me? What do you mean?"

"You know. You have to ride the 'L,' walk around at night."

He meant he would get money by robbing people like me. It was a subtle attempt to assert his dominance. But that was, as they say in poker, a "tell."

In the hospital, patients lose their freedom; they are no longer in control of their environment. As a response they will occasionally do things to reassert their independence. A subtle fact about hospitals is that to ensure smooth running, the hospital must infantilize patients in small ways—the hospital gown, tests scheduled at certain hours, strict mealtimes, and occasionally a patronizing remark by the staff.

A patient may rebel in his or her own way, by adopting an argumentative or demanding posture. Women may become flirtatious with the staff, men sexually suggestive. These are signs of weakness rather than strength, and at least to some degree, they are understandable. In fact, doctors and nurses who become patients are among the worst offenders in attempting to regain control. They are more aware than most of what is happening to them in the hospital.

Jeffrey's attempt to scare me told me that actually he was the one who was scared. Right then, I knew I could make eye contact with him, something very few people did outside the hospital. And looking into those eyes, I did not see a vicious street gangbanger, but a frightened twenty-three-year-old who knew he was quite sick. I did not linger on the subject of his drug use.

"Well, Jeffrey, you won't be on my ward much longer. You will be going to surgery pretty soon."

He trembled slightly. "You think it will be OK, Doc?" I knew when he asked that question he was indeed no different from any other scared young man in the hospital.

"Yeah, I do. But you have to shake that habit."

My reassurance allowed him to revert to type. He nodded and his scowl reappeared. The conversation was over.

The next morning something unexpected happened. In the cafeteria I was approached by one of the women from "environmental services" whose job it was to clean the ward. I knew her casually; she was a friendly but taciturn middle-aged woman who always greeted me with a smile. Every Christmas, she gave me a religious card.

"Dr. Franklin, do you think Jeffrey is going to be OK?" I knew that as a woman of faith working in the hospital, she was concerned with the welfare of every patient, but for her to approach me and ask about a particular patient by first name was unusual.

"I think he will, Mrs. Andrews." The fact they had the same last name didn't occur to me. Then, without prompting, she explained the cause of her concern. It was something of a shock.

"Jeffrey is my son."

A faint air of resignation was in her voice. It must have been difficult for this churchgoing woman to acknowledge what her son had become and see the state he was in. But the most powerful force in the world is maternal love. She was deeply worried and so I tried my best to console her.

"Mrs. Andrews, I'm sure he will be OK."

That afternoon, Jeffrey sat on the open ward when Mrs. Andrews walked right by him, no more than three feet away. From a distance, I watched as she passed him without saying a word, although she did acknowledge him by staring directly in his face. Men's lives had undoubtedly been threatened for lesser stares at Jeffrey. Yet he could not confront her gaze for more than an instant before bowing his head in shame. She shook her head ruefully and left the ward while he glanced around to see if anyone had noticed.

From the corner of the ward I witnessed the entire mini-drama, although he did not realize it.

The next day he was transferred to surgery. I didn't see him again during that hospitalization. I was told he had his skin grafts and went home without complications.

About a year later, I saw Jeffrey briefly. I was doing a consult in the trauma unit and he walked through with some of his fellow gang members to visit a friend who had been involved in a gang firefight, with several nonlethal bullet wounds to show for it. He and his friends were outfitted in what appeared to be gang colors (a type of uniform that does draw respect) and he walked through the ward with a swagger and a sneer. He made no effort to conceal his contempt for the doctors and nurses taking care of his friend.

His eyes met mine for a second; I could tell he recognized me, but he made no effort to acknowledge me. I earned the same withering glare as everyone else, and I averted my gaze quickly. The brief reunion was over. I thought that would be the last time I would ever see Jeffrey.

I was wrong.

All of this transpired in the early 1980s, when it was common knowledge in the medical community that drug use involving dirty needles could cause skin abscesses, blood infections, and hepatitis. But the AIDS virus, HIV, had just been isolated, and while the association between drug use and AIDS was suspected, dirty needle use was still not recognized as a major risk factor. That would become known just a few short years later. As we later learned, the drug users of the late 1970s and early '80s like Jeffrey were at an incredibly high risk of contracting AIDS from their needle use.

Flash forward twenty years to the early 2000s. One day on my way to the ICU, I walked through the dialysis ward of the hospital and saw a chart with the name Jeff Andrews. The names of certain patients stay with you, sometimes for decades. That one had stayed with me. My first thought was that it couldn't possibly be the same Jeff Andrews, but I had to know. I checked the date of birth on the chart. The patient was in his early forties, the same age Jeffrey would have been. I went to the room number on the chart. (These were the days before confidentiality laws made finding a patient's room much harder.)

In that room, an old man was in bed, sleeping lightly. He was certainly much older than Jeffrey would have been. He was bald, and even though he was sleeping his hands and face trembled involuntarily. The sign above his bed said he was blind. Next to his bed was a wheelchair, but there was no sign of the type of walking cane blind patients use. It appeared he was unable to walk by himself.

My first thought was that I had misread the room number. I was about to go back to the chart to find out where Jeff Andrews was when I stopped and looked at the old man's legs. There were skin grafts, in the exact places where Jeffrey had his skin infections twenty years ago. I looked closely at the face on the old man. There was a facial tic and spittle running off his lower lip—certainly no fierce visage. But his face told the story: there was no question the old man was Jeffrey. How could that be? This man looked to be eighty years old. And it was clear to me he was close to death.

I found the resident responsible for the cases on the ward and asked about Jeffrey. I didn't mention my connection; when I first met Jeffrey this resident would have been in grade school. He wouldn't understand.

The resident told me Jeffrey did indeed have end-stage AIDS, contracted from needle use. Infections from HIV had blinded him and he was on the dialysis ward because his kidneys were destroyed. He was demented, unable to feed himself or use the bathroom, and wheelchair-bound. In the twenty years since I had last seen Jeffrey, he had aged more than a lifetime. The resident told me that Jeffrey had three months to live, six at most. Having cared for hundreds of AIDS patients, I knew the resident's prognosis was overly optimistic.

I went back to see Jeffrey, who was now awake. The nurses had him sitting in a chair and were spoon-feeding him. The feared gangbanger who once terrorized the West Side of Chicago had grits dribbling down his chin into his lap. I did not say anything to him and he probably couldn't hear me or understand anyway. Ironically, there was no point in making eye contact, that same eye contact that once made people shiver. For the first time, I noticed his facial resemblance to his mother.

The next day I went to environmental services and looked up a woman whom I had known for many years, since the days she was a young trainee. Now she was a supervisor of environmental services.

"Ms. Logan, does Henrietta Andrews still work here?'

She gave me a surprised look.

"Mrs. Andrews? Dr. Franklin, she hasn't been here for ten years. She retired when she got cancer of the womb. She died about four years ago. I remember her homegoing." Her funeral. "It was beautiful."

"Thanks, Ms. Logan."

It was sad to hear that Mrs. Andrews was gone. But in a way I was thankful. She would never have wanted to see her son the way he was now.

And it turned out I was right about how long Jeffrey had to live. Ten days later, he was dead.

6

A BLACK MAN IN DALLAS ON THE DAY JFK WAS ASSASSINATED

"From Dallas, Texas, the flash, apparently official:
President Kennedy died at 1 PM central standard time,
2:00 eastern standard time, some thirty-eight minutes ago."

—WALTER CRONKITE

CW WAS ONE of the nicest patients I ever took care of. A truly good person. He's almost certainly dead today; he was in his late forties back in the early 1980s and he had a failing heart even then. He had been in the hospital for over a month, because in those days people with chronic heart infections had to stay in the hospital to get antibiotic treatment. Today, he would get his antibiotics as an outpatient.

I would see him every day, and for someone with a bad heart he was unfailingly cheerful; he never felt sorry for himself. He was a black man from Texas, with a thick Texas drawl. He sounded something like Tommy Lee Jones. I imagined him wearing a cowboy hat outside the hospital, though I never saw one among his belongings. He was small, no more than five foot five, with a round face and a perpetually swollen belly from retained fluid, a result of his heart failure. One other notable thing about him: he had no teeth. Each day when we visited him on rounds, he greeted the whole team with that drawl and toothless grin, "How are y'all doctors today?" And unlike some, he really cared about the answer.

He greeted the nurses the same way. And in the days of open wards, he would socialize with all the other patients. He'd help the old men to the bathroom, and he would try to counsel the young heroin users, even the many who were gang members. They never paid him any mind; to them he was just another foolish old man. But he was never put off by them.

"Them young bucks, they'll learn. If they stay alive." He was right, of course.

His heart failure was the result of a chronic bacterial infection of a heart valve. Over time, the infection prevented his heart from pumping blood effectively, and fluid backed up into his legs and abdomen, like a sink with an open faucet and a drain that wouldn't close all the way.

His condition happened to be a rarity—a "fascinoma," as we called uncommon cases. The bacterium that infected his heart was quite unusual; it almost never invaded a heart valve. The organism was found in the mouth, related to his teeth, or lack thereof.

As he explained it to me, he was unable to afford a dentist, so when he had a bad tooth he simply pulled it himself. I asked him how he did it.

He grinned proudly and said, "With pliers." When he told me that, I shuddered, because for the first time I understood that his toothless grin represented a lot of pain.

Unfortunately, in pulling one of those teeth, he seeded his bloodstream with bacteria, and a particularly indolent organism had lodged on his heart valve. Over time, it had eaten away the valve. A long course of antibiotics, followed by surgery, was the only chance he could be cured. Otherwise fluid would continue to back up, and when it reached his lungs he would suffocate slowly.

Because his infection was so unusual, I decided to present his case to the experts at the university hospital in a medical conference. No one had ever seen a case exactly like CW's. At some point I told them about the pliers and how he had acquired his infection. The fact that CW had pulled his teeth with pliers proved a source of no small amusement to the men in the white coats. There were jokes and disparaging remarks all around the elegant wood-paneled conference room about this simple man from Texas who had no access to a dentist and no other recourse. To these fancy doctors, CW was not a real person; he was just another case, and a humorous one at that. Pulling your teeth with pliers. Who does that?

I took umbrage at the supercilious attitude of the group, but what could I say? To remark on their callousness would be embarrassing—and besides, it would serve little purpose. The human disconnect between these "experts" in their case conference and the poor patient was too wide a gap to bridge. Many of them were probably empathetic people as medical students, but they had lost their empathy for people like CW long ago. Their detachment was merely the way they were expected to act in the rarified air of the university medical center. Happens with doctors all the time. Not to all of them, but to many.

This was not the first time I had encountered this attitude of disdain for the patient among physicians. It would be tempting to simplify it as a racial thing or a rich/poor thing. But it was neither, as illustrated by this next example.

Once, I sat in a conference with a different set of experts at a different university hospital. The patient—actually, she was referred to as a "case"—was a middle-aged woman who had undergone a routine knee replacement. Unexpectedly, the surgery went badly and she suffered a devastating complication. Even as the conference was going on, she was in shock and close to death. The group of experts regarded this woman's complication rather cavalierly. There was little sense of concern that this recently healthy patient, probably someone's wife and mother, was now dying.

In fact, she was indeed someone's wife and mother.

I realized that the patient they were discussing was actually the mother of a good friend of mine, a girl I had known since I was a boy. (I made the logical connection because I knew that her mother had gone to that hospital for surgery and had suffered a life-threatening complication, and now I was hearing about a case of a woman her age fitting the description perfectly.) Now I knew her mother would be dead soon, and I felt uneasy and more than a little contemptuous about the lack of concern by the doctors in that elegant paneled room.

I thought of her daughter, with whom I went to grade school. She wasn't there and didn't understand exactly what happened to her mother, but she knew how sick she was. Since I wasn't directly connected to her mother's case, and it was a different hospital, it was left to others to explain the nature of the complication to my friend. My friend would not even be aware that I knew about the case.

The disconnect between the vibrant woman I had known and liked for years and the callousness of how these doctors discussed "the case" bothered me. Like CW, she was not a real patient to them. Disgusted, I walked out before it was over; I couldn't listen any longer. I never told her daughter about the conference.

That way doctors identify patients as "this week's case conference subject," oblivious to the real, live people in distress, was something I saw many other times. But when I heard these doctors discussing CW, and my mind drifted back to how a different group of doctors had referred to my mother's friend in the same callous fashion, I said nothing as I left the wood-paneled room.

A strange feeling came over me when I came back to the ward CW was on, and I felt compelled to go over and talk with him. Nothing important, just chat. Perhaps it was guilt; perhaps I just wanted to make contact. Like always, he was glad to see me.

"How's it going, Doc?" That Texas drawl and the toothless smile.

"CW, I'm curious, where in Texas are you from?

"Dallas. Dallas, Texas." He said it proudly, as any Texan would.

"What kind of work did you do, CW?"

"I used to paint houses and buildings. I even did some painting at the Adolphus Hotel."

You could tell he was proud of working on the ritziest hotel in Dallas. Meanwhile, I did some quick mental math.

"CW, were you in Dallas when President Kennedy was killed?"

"Doc, I wasn't just in Dallas. I was helping paint Parkland Hospital that day."

I had been a student of the assassination for years and CW was the first person I ever met who was actually in Dallas on November 22, 1963. Not only was he in Dallas but at Parkland, the hospital to which the mortally wounded president was brought.

"What was it like? What do you remember, CW?"

"All I remember, Doc, is that you didn't want to be a black man in Dallas that day."

I will never forget CW.

7

RIB TIPS AND HOMEGOINGS

"Let death . . . be daily before your eyes . . . and you will never entertain any abject thought, nor too eagerly covet anything."

—EPICTETUS

FOR PHYSICIANS, NOTHING is harder than losing a patient. That's true even of patients you have never encountered before they were hospitalized. But it's especially true of those patients who were with you for years, whom you came to know, and with whom you had the privilege of becoming friends.

Every year, Mr. Baker made Thanksgiving especially memorable for my family and me. He was one of my clinic patients—one of my favorites, in fact, for reasons to become clear. When I first met him, his blood pressure was extremely high and he had mild diabetes. In the hospital, the doctors told him he would have to take a lot of medications when he went home to bring his blood pressure down. But they didn't do a great job of following up, no one was in charge of his care, and eventually he wound up in my clinic by chance.

The approach to patients who are admitted with high blood pressure has been one of my pet peeves at every hospital where I have worked. When the blood pressure is high enough for the patient to be admitted to the hospital, the diagnosis is known by a variety of terms—hypertensive urgency, hypertensive emergency, hypertensive crisis—although it's often hard to fathom the distinction. In all cases, we're talking about extremely high blood pressure that threatens the patient's heart, kidneys, or brain.

Some patients must have their blood pressure normalized immediately, but usually it's just a matter of getting control over a period of several days to several weeks. All too often what happens is the opposite of what should happen. Instead of bringing down the blood pressure gradually and making sure the patient gets prompt outpatient follow-up, the doctors in the hospital bring the blood pressure down quickly—sometimes too quickly, which can be dangerous. Then they ignore the follow-up that is critical to controlling the patient's chronic high blood pressure and optimizing his or her long-term health.

That's what happened to Mr. Baker. He came to the emergency room because of pain in his hip, and incidentally his blood pressure was found to be 205/120. He spent three days in the hospital while the doctors gave him all sorts of blood pressure medications, which lowered his blood pressure too fast, and he had to be sent to the intensive care unit. He recovered, but when he was discharged from the hospital he was given a clinic appointment three months down the line with a doctor who had never taken care of him. When he eventually ended up in my clinic, his blood pressure was close to where it had been when he had first come to the hospital three months before. A lot of time and money expended for very little benefit. The worst of American medicine at work.

Over the next six months, we worked to control Mr. Baker's blood pressure and his diabetes. I would see him in the clinic once every ten weeks. He was still bothered by severe pain in his hip, but despite this, he was invariably cheerful and had a smile for everyone in the clinic. Good follow-up, not medical genius, is what kept him out of the hospital.

One day he came to clinic with a box of food. It smelled delicious. I asked him if it was his lunch.

"No, Doc. It's for you."

"You're kidding. What is it?"

"Rib tips. The best ribs you ever tasted. I guarantee you. Try them."

Ribs are pretty messy, so I figured I should wait until clinic was over. But the smell of those ribs was irresistible. I *had* to try them.

"Maybe I'll just try one."

Mr. Baker chuckled.

The rib tip I tried tasted even better than it smelled. They *were* the best ribs I had ever eaten. I ate the entire box and spent the next ten minutes washing my hands so I could finish up clinic.

"Mr. Baker, where did you get those ribs?"

"I make them."

"Really?"

"Doc, I've got a rib joint out in Maywood. People come from all over. Even Mississippi. If you like them, I can bring you in a box every time I come to clinic."

"That would be great."

I was probably violating something in the Hippocratic canon when I increased the frequency of his visits from every ten weeks to every nine weeks. It was certainly a conflict of interest on my part, but it did mean an extra box of ribs every year.

There was a minor problem in that everyone in the clinic could smell the ribs when Mr. Baker came to clinic. It didn't take long for people to figure out I was the one getting those ribs. Everyone wanted to try them. Occasionally, I would let another doctor or nurse try one, not so much out of generosity but as a way of showing off.

He's my patient—taste how good these ribs are.

The perk got better. One afternoon in mid-November, Mr. Baker came to clinic with his customary gift. He was doing well clinically, except for his hip pain. He had developed a noticeable limp. I took an X-ray and it showed he had severe degenerative arthritis; his joint was bone on bone, with no cushioning cartilage. I told him his hip looked bad, that he might need surgery, and we would reevaluate him after the first of the year.

"Whatever you think, Doc. By the way, Thanksgiving is next week. You know I smoke a real nice turkey. I'd like to give you one. Can you meet me at the hospital here around 1 PM on Thursday?"

"Sure, Mr. Baker."

Thanksgiving was my favorite holiday, and I always made sure to have the day off. In the morning, I loved watching the Macy's parade with my kids. But that year, as soon as it was over, I told my wife I had to go down to the hospital. It was sort of an emergency. When I got there Mr. Baker was waiting in the lobby with a completely cooked turkey.

"Just pop it in the oven to warm it up, Doc. It'll be great eating."

It was. We had never had a turkey like that. And the leftovers were great, too.

Mr. Baker made our Thanksgiving rendezvous an annual tradition. For the next five years, my family had two turkeys for our Thanksgiving meal: the one my wife made and the one Mr. Baker had generously cooked for us. I offered him money, but he never accepted it.

"Come on, Doc. I couldn't take your money."

Mr. Baker came regularly to the clinic. His blood pressure and diabetes were under control, and he brought ribs with him to every clinic visit and a smoked turkey at Thanksgiving. I never figured out how, with all that good cooking, he managed to keep his weight down.

There was one problem.

It was that hip. Over time, the pain was getting worse, as was his limp. We tried managing it with pain medications and physical therapy, to no avail. After about a year, I figured he needed a hip replacement and referred him to our orthopedic surgeons, who agreed he was a candidate for surgery.

The problem was that County Hospital did not do many elective hip surgeries. There were too many trauma cases, not enough operating rooms, and too few anesthesiologists and orthopedic surgeons. No one came right out and said that; it would not look good politically to admit that County didn't do elective hip surgery. So they used what's called "the strategy of the long wait."

People would be scheduled for surgery in a long waiting list, four to six months. Eventually, most people would drop out or be lost to follow-up. Those who managed to wait it out would then be put off for another four to six months. That way, there was always a waiting list and very few patients ever got the elective surgery. Sort of like the old Soviet Union.

Mr. Baker was put on the waiting list, and every time he came to clinic, I checked on his position. He never made any headway. So after another year, he and I both came to the realization that he would never get an artificial hip at County. Meanwhile, he soldiered bravely through the pain.

I decided that we would try the university hospital. I called a friend, an orthopedic surgeon on the university hospital staff. He told me he would like to operate on Mr. Baker but his hands were tied, because Mr. Baker did not have insurance the hospital would accept. But he told us to keep trying; the hospital might be able to make arrangements.

For another year and a half, it became a standing joke between Mr. Baker and me. What was it going to take for him to get surgery? By this time, he was using a cane and getting around was quite difficult, but he maintained his good humor. "Whenever it happens, it happens," he said. I had few patients who were that understanding.

Finally, after four years of Thanksgiving turkeys, I got a call from my orthopedist friend. He could see Mr. Baker in his office and evaluate him for surgery. I had Mr. Baker come in right away to see me to make sure all his medical problems were in check, and sent him with his X-rays to see my friend (at the time we had no way to send X-rays electronically). This might be our only chance.

My friend called and told me Mr. Baker had one of the worst hips he had ever seen. He would definitely need surgery, but since he was a char-ity patient it could not be scheduled at the university hospital for another eight weeks. Just the same, it looked like Mr. Baker would finally get his surgery and a new hip.

Eight excruciatingly painful weeks went by before Mr. Baker's surgery. If this were a movie, the unhappy ending to the story would be that the surgery went badly.

But the surgery went fine. Better than expected.

Mr. Baker got a new hip without any complications. The orthopedic surgeon called me proudly to tell me the news, said he would be sending Mr. Baker home in a day or two, and asked if I would do medical follow-up in a month.

That was wonderful news, and a month later Mr. Baker was seeing me in the clinic. He was so happy. He was walking much better, and had no pain. Everything was going great.

"Thanks so much, Doc. I feel great. I can't thank you enough. You know, next month is Thanksgiving. See you then."

We both knew it would be time for a smoked turkey.

On the appointed day, I met Mr. Baker and we talked for a while.

"Doc, I'm doing great. I'm taking longer and longer walks. Three blocks yesterday. I can't believe it. It's amazing. Here you go, Doc."

He presented me with my smoked turkey.

"It's an especially good one this year, Doc. When do you want to see me again in clinic?"

"Mr. Baker, let's try for right after the holidays. First week in January."

"Sounds good. Happy Thanksgiving, Doc. Have a good Christmas and a happy new year. I can't thank you enough. See you soon."

"See you next year, Mr. Baker. Thanks again."

"No, thank *you*, Doc! Enjoy the turkey." As he said that, he smiled and walked away.

It was the last time I saw him.

On his scheduled appointment day in January, he did not show up on time. I saw some other patients first and thought he was delayed because of the bad weather. But after I had seen my last patient, he had still not arrived. I gave him another ten minutes and then decided to call him.

Right before I picked up the phone, I smelled a familiar aroma in the clinic hallway. A young man knocked on the door of my examining room and entered with a box of ribs.

"Dr. Franklin, I'm Mr. Baker's son. I know he would have wanted you to have these. I made them."

"Where is your dad?"

"He passed."

"When?"

"Right before Christmas."

'What happened?"

The young man began crying.

"He was doing fine and he had just come in from a walk. He went into the kitchen and just collapsed. We called the paramedics and they took him to the hospital near our home, but they told us he was dead by the time he got there. They said there was nothing they could do."

My heart sank.

"I'm so sorry. Is there anything I can do?"

"No, Doc. I know how much he liked you. And you really took care of him. We're closing up the rib shack, but I just wanted to drop these off for you." He left before I could say anything else.

I will never know exactly what happened, but if I had to guess, Mr. Baker had suffered a heart attack. I think that while he waited five years for a new hip, he completely restricted his activity. When he finally had the surgery and recovered, he started increasing his physical activity to a level his heart couldn't tolerate. Sadly, three short months was only as long as he got to enjoy the new hip that he had gone through so much for and waited so long to get.

I lost my appetite. Rather than eat the ribs then, I took them home with me to enjoy later. Mr. Baker's son was not quite the cook his dad was. But that wasn't really the reason the ribs didn't taste quite as good as they had in the past.

I wasn't able to go to Mr. Baker's funeral, but I have attended services honoring other longtime patients. Many of these patients were black and poor, so it meant traveling into unfamiliar neighborhoods, and I was often one of the few white people there. Sometimes the *only* white person there. Being the only white face in certain settings draws attention, just like being the only black face in others.

Even so, it gave me peace of mind to see my patients and their families one last time. The services were unlike those I was used to. Occasionally, the family of the deceased would even ask me to say a few words.

Of all the patient funerals—or "homegoings," as they were often called—I ever attended, the most memorable was that of Mr. Buckles. (The "homegoing" is a festive funeral rite that's culturally ingrained in the African American community; its roots reach back four centuries to the Dahomeans of Benin and the Yoruba of Nigeria, West Africa. They are thought to have brought the ritual from ancient Egypt.) Mr. Buckles was my patient for twenty-five years, and I also took care of his wife and several of his adult children. The last few years of his life he was quite ill, and he visited the clinic frequently. Everyone at the clinic knew him.

When he died, his family told me how much they appreciated everything the hospital and I had done for him, and they made a point of asking me to come to his funeral. It was an honor.

It turned out that Mr. Buckles's funeral was in one of the roughest neighborhoods on the South Side. On the appointed morning, I drove down to the funeral service. Not surprisingly, mine was the only white face to be seen for city blocks. Like other South Side neighborhoods, there were pockets of respectable middle-class homes right next to boarded-up storefronts with gang graffiti on the windows, but you could tell it had the air of violence.

It was a cold, quiet winter morning. Mr. Buckles was popular in his neighborhood and it was a crowded funeral, so I had to park about a block away. Experience had taught me that most gangbangers did not come out at that time of day, so I felt reasonably safe. Even so I remained alert, out of habit. As I neared the church, the street was filled with impeccably dressed funeral-goers, some of whom I recognized, one or two of whom may have even been in my clinic. Once inside, I felt the warm, familiar feeling of a reverent congregation. It was quite comforting.

The beautiful service was long and emotional, as many funerals in black neighborhoods are. I wanted to stay for the whole service, but since I had to return to the hospital for my clinic, I left early. The spirituality I had experienced in the church removed all my trepidation as I walked back to my car.

Driving to the hospital after the service, I had a good feeling about Mr. Buckles and I reminisced about what a wonderful patient he had been. I recalled him telling me what a good athlete he'd been in high school fifty years ago. He was a track and football star, something you would never have imagined if you had seen him during the last few years of his life: old and obese, with heart trouble. I thought back to one of our conversations.

"If we raced, Doc, I would have left you in the dust."

"Not anymore you wouldn't."

"No, but back then I could spot you fifty yards and beat you in the hundred."

My guess is that he could have.

I was half an hour late getting back to clinic, which was unusual for me. Besides that, I was better dressed than usual, wearing a nice button-down shirt and khakis instead of my customary jeans. The nurses, used to me being prompt and casually dressed, knew something was up.

"Where you been, Dr. Franklin?"

"I was at Mr. Buckles's homegoing."

Some of them hadn't heard he had died.

"How was the funeral?"

"It was really nice. Glad I went."

"Where was it?"

"It was in South Chicago. Church was just off Marquette."

The nurses, who were all black, stared at me. They knew better than I that it was a dangerous neighborhood, somewhere most white people never ventured.

"Dr. Franklin, that's *the 'hood*. We don't even go around there."

I shrugged and said, "You know, it didn't seem so bad. I had no problems."

"Nobody bothered you?"

"Not at all."

"Is that the way you were dressed?"

"Yes, why?"

"They thought you were a cop."

8

OF LITTLE GREEN MEN
AND IMAGINARY HIGHWAYS

"To alcohol, the cause of, and solution to,
all of life's problems."

—HOMER SIMPSON

I N THE HOSPITAL, alcohol use is a huge issue. When a patient has a
drinking problem, the physician's job is to provide counsel and follow
up in future clinic visits by asking them if they have stopped drinking.
Some patients do and will tell their doctor so. Some don't, and they pre-
varicate about it. By far the most imaginative answer I ever heard was
when I asked one of my long-term patients, "Well, Mrs. Thomas, have you
stopped drinking?"

She didn't break stride. "Have they stopped making it? When they stop
making it, I'll stop drinking."

While I would have preferred that she stop drinking, this sort of admi-
rable candor was the next best thing.

Alcohol certainly caused its share of problems for patients at County Hospital, and does everywhere for that matter—cirrhosis, heart disease, accidents, trauma; neurologic, dietary, and metabolic problems. Despite this, patients continue to "quaff this kind nepenthe" in search of respite, as Edgar Allan Poe, no slouch when it came to drinking, so aptly described it.

Our view of alcoholism today is far different than it was forty years ago. Movies and television no longer portray the "lovable drunk." Society, at least outside of the fraternity party, frowns on public intoxication. Back then, though, the problems caused by alcohol were ubiquitous in hospitals, and few people did anything to address them proactively. At County, with the exception of the occasional well-meaning social worker or young physician, most of the staff accepted with resignation the problem of alcoholism in our patients.

In a hospital with a thousand inpatients, of whom perhaps 10 percent had some problem with alcohol, a weekly inpatient Alcoholics Anonymous meeting rarely drew as many as ten referrals from the staff. Not too impressive. The director of the AA program, a former alcoholic himself, often asked me about the lack of referrals. There was nothing I could do but shrug my shoulders. Today, the incentive to discharge patients quickly means that few patients are in the hospital long enough to benefit from an inpatient AA program.

———————————

On the hospital wards, the most dramatic manifestation of alcohol was delirium tremens, or as they were more commonly known, DTs. Alcohol is a habit-forming drug, and DTs are a form of withdrawal that occurs when the drug is unavailable. DTs are, in fact, the most vivid and violent form of alcohol withdrawal.

When ingested, alcohol creates a tolerance in the human body, and when the person stops drinking his or her body reacts violently. A hangover the morning after a night of drinking is a withdrawal reaction, albeit one that is comparatively mild. Since a hangover is a form of drug withdrawal, despite all the touted home remedies, there is only one reliable cure: more alcohol. This has been known for centuries as "hair of the dog," an expression that derived from the practice of treating the bite of a rabid dog by placing hair from the dog in the bite wound.

Treating a hangover with more alcohol, while immediately effective, is obviously counterproductive in the long run. Since alcohol is so cheap and access so easy in our culture, most alcoholics can just go out and get more alcohol and repeat the cycle. The longer one drinks, the more severe the withdrawal when one stops (not to mention the habituation and long-term damage). And the withdrawal becomes more and more violent as time goes on. This is due to the complex interaction of brain cells firing off in an excited fashion. Those who drink will notice that after the initial inebriation, the effect of too much alcohol is to induce sleep, but the sleep that results is usually fitful and not the normal deep sleep. In medical terms, alcohol disrupts the crucial rapid eye movement (REM) sleep.

True severe DTs are not as common in the hospital as they once were. Even many experienced physicians have never seen a case. It generally takes two to three months of daily consumption of large amounts of alcohol to create the conditions under which DTs would result from sudden abstinence. It was more prevalent decades ago and was generally familiar in popular culture, with vivid portrayals by Ray Milland in the movie *The Lost Weekend* and Jack Lemmon in *Days of Wine and Roses*. Those were the rare exceptions to the "lovable drunk" archetype.

Most severe DTs are the result of forced abstinence. A heavy drinker hospitalized for surgery or with trauma—commonly an alcohol-related automobile accident—in the course of several days without access to alcohol would develop DTs. One of the most common scenarios was the jail patient transferred to the hospital. The person would be arrested, usually for some minor alcohol-related offense, couldn't make bail, and after four days in jail would start developing DTs.

Severe DTs are a medical emergency, and if untreated or poorly treated the patient can die as a result. (Even those who survive often die later in life of liver disease or trauma in which alcohol is involved.) Affected patients develop tremors and become confused, then agitated, then violent. They sweat profusely, their blood pressure and pulse shoot way up, and they hallucinate. Often they imagine insects crawling all over their bodies. Sometimes the hallucinations are visual; in *The Lost Weekend*, Ray Milland sees imaginary rodents, and in *Days of Wine and Roses*, Jack Lemmon sees a little green man.

For a time, every inhibition is removed. I saw patients in DTs spit, curse, and call nurses and physicians the worst, most vulgar names imaginable. When the DTs were over, those same patients were quite often not only friendly but gentle and accommodating. They had no memory of the aberrant behavior exhibited only a few days before.

The preferred treatment for DTs is to give the patient a cross-tolerant sedative drug, usually something like Librium, Valium, or a related compound. For advanced DTs, the sedative must be given intravenously with large amounts of fluid, since the patient is unable to follow commands to swallow and will likely spit out pills. Also, the patient must generally be in restraints, because of the likelihood of exhibiting violence. DTs are one of the most common reasons for a patient to be restrained.

———

Though DTs are a serious, life-threatening emergency, I treated them enough over the years to find that there was an element of dark humor to them. This is not meant to demean the patients in any way, merely to point out that health care personnel, like the police or military, develop their own brand of humor as a way of coping. DTs could provide a fertile source. The doctor treating Jack Lemmon's character in the movie certainly might have been smiling to himself over his patient's little green man.

One of the first signs that a patient may be going into DTs is confabulation, when he or she creates and relates a false memory—one that often involves the doctor. I was amazed at how consistent this phenomenon could be.

DTs do not respect race, religion, or economic status. (Women, though, for some reason seem far less prone to DTs.) When I worked as a student at the university hospital, I saw an extremely successful, white bank vice president who was confabulating before going into DTs. Although I had never met him before, the bank VP described to me quite lucidly, and in great detail, how the week before I'd had breakfast with him at the Union League Club, one of the most posh meeting places in Chicago and no doubt one of his breakfast haunts. In his mind, this shared meal had actually happened. He "remembered" it quite specifically: I had steak and eggs and a large glass of orange juice; we left together before I went to work at the hospital. In reality, I had never been to the Union League Club in my life.

About a year later, back at County, I saw a man about the same age who was black and did not have a steady job. I had never met him before either, but he confabulated about a similar breakfast meeting. He and I also had dined last week, not at the Union League Club but at a greasy spoon on Madison Street, likely a place he frequented. This time I did not have steak and eggs but grits, sausage, and coffee. We left together before I went to work at the hospital. Two people, both with the same confabulation altered only by their circumstances, before they lapsed into DTs. It is truly amazing how the human mind works.

Once the patient is in full-blown DTs and the hallucinations take over, he is no longer aware of the reality around him. The hallucinations are not always little green men or rodents or pink elephants, but no matter what they are, they are vivid. Once we had two patients in beds next to each other in an open ward, both in DTs, restrained, hallucinating, and shouting at the top of their lungs. At first they were oblivious of each other. Then one of them imagined himself in a car accident on the Dan Ryan Expressway, the busy highway leading into Chicago. He started yelling to no one in particular, "DAMN, WHY DID YOU HIT MY CAR? WHAT DID YOU HIT MY CAR FOR?"

Suddenly, quite unexpectedly, the other patient left whatever dream state he was in and began answering him. Now he was in the same hallucination. He was also on the Dan Ryan.

"I DIDN'T HIT YOUR CAR! YOU HIT MY CAR!"

"I'LL GET MY TIRE IRON. TAKE CARE OF YOU."

"I'LL GET MY PIECE."

Their actual exchange included considerably more profanity, but they had somehow created a simulated traffic encounter, complete with threats, all of this being played out on the ward.

A week later, these two men, who in their hallucinations had been threatening to kill each other on the shoulder of the highway, recovered from the DTs and became fast friends on the ward. Perhaps they became drinking buddies when they left the hospital.

———————

As mentioned before, one of the most important management aspects of DTs is patient restraint. Straitjackets, like the one Jack Lemmon wore in *Days of Wine and Roses*, are a thing of the past, but restraining a patient— essentially, tying them to a bed with strong cloth—is still heart-wrenching to watch and even more difficult to order or carry out. By doing so, you take away the patient's last vestige of freedom. Every nurse and doctor has personal feelings and a philosophy about the process. Some are aggressive about restraining patients, especially if they are difficult to control. Others with a stronger sense of civil liberties shy away from using restraints. But every nurse and physician has had to resort to them at some point.

Technically, going by the book, the indications for restraining patients are when they represent a physical harm to themselves or others. This is often a judgment call, and there is a lot of latitude in that judgment. The ability to restrain a patient is one of the demonstrations of the power care-givers have over patients. Often it is the ultimate demonstration. Next to jail, the hospital carries the potential of the greatest threat to the average citizen's civil liberties.

The patient going into DTs can turn violent quickly; the surges of adrenaline they experience often give them great strength. They *must* be restrained. Indeed, one of my worst hospital episodes was over a failure to do just that.

We had a patient on the open ward on the third floor who was develop-ing DTs. Although I was the supervising resident, I was not the managing resident for this patient. His managing residents were strong proponents of civil liberties; they believed restraints were an unwarranted coercion, a tyrannical restriction of the patient's freedom. No matter that the patient was hallucinating and extremely agitated. When he started seeing bugs and picking at imaginary insects crawling all over his arms, he suddenly pulled out his intravenous line. Because his residents had done nothing to restrain him, he climbed over his bedrails and began running down the ward, attempting to escape his imaginary torment.

He made it to the fire escape and pushed open the emergency exit, which triggered the fire alarm. That, in turn, automatically summoned the fire department. The patient stood on the fire escape, and rather than running down the stairs, he lingered for what seemed an eternity, threat-ening to jump. It took about fifteen minutes until the fire crew arrived, and during that time we tried to talk him off the fire escape, to no avail. At any moment, he could have decided to jump, and we were essentially powerless to stop him.

Finally the Chicago Fire Department arrived, and a gruff battalion chief came to the ward. He assessed the situation, calmly deployed some men on the ground below the fire escape, and was able to talk the man back in.

He asked what happened and who was in charge. I sheepishly told him I was. He was stern but friendly, and told me to take care that it did not happen again.

While I was duly chastised, the residents in charge of the case were not present when the fire chief was there, and the gravity of the situation did not impress them. They remained staunch civil libertarians. They put another intravenous line in the patient and sedated him (which they refused to recognize as simply a different way of infringing on the patient's liberties), but they remained adamant they would not restrain the patient. To them, it was the principle of the thing. The nurses were not happy; I was not happy as the senior resident, but I received no support from my immediate superior, the chief resident, who was politically sympathetic to the managing residents. I was admonished that to restrain the patient would be a form of "medical fascism." I attempted to point out the silliness of such a view in light of the fact the patient had nearly jumped off the fire escape, but I was overruled.

In the middle of the night, about four hours later, I was on the ward alone when the patient's sedation wore off. This time, he bit through his intravenous line, spewing blood all over, and jumped the bedrails once again. Now, intimately familiar with the path to the fire escape, he ran down the hall and again forced the door open. Fire alarm, fire department summoned. This time the only thing that kept him from jumping was the fact that his hospital trousers kept falling down. It bought us the fifteen minutes until the arrival of the same battalion chief, and he relieved the situation masterfully a second time. A real pro.

There was a general commotion on the ward as people filtered in. However, the battalion chief went straight for the familiar face, which happened to be me. This time he was flushed, much sterner, and not so friendly as he'd been before.

"Listen. If this happens again, if I have to come back for any reason, any reason, *you* are going to be in big trouble."

I was uncertain if he was referring to administrative trouble, physical trouble (he was a big guy), or both, and I was in no position to ascertain the specific nature of the threat. There was no excuse available. I was reduced to a meek "Yes, sir."

When the battalion chief left, I went right to the chief resident and the managing residents, who seemingly had been quite happy to let me take the full force of the wrath of the fire department. Fortunately, I was physically bigger than any of the civil libertarians, and I issued the only physical threat of my medical career. I looked each one in the eye.

"If you guys don't restrain that patient, one of you is going to need a hospital bed."

They finally restrained the patient. No more evening forays onto the fire escape, no more visits from the fire department.

A patient in severe DTs should always be restrained.

9

POISONS: KGB UMBRELLAS, THE FIRST RICIN SURVIVOR, AND A SUICIDAL BIOCHEMIST

"If you poison us, do we not die?"

—WILLIAM SHAKESPEARE, *THE MERCHANT OF VENICE*

P OISONS, SO UBIQUITOUS in our environment, have played a significant role in literature and history. Romeo and Juliet, Socrates, Cleopa-
tra, and Marilyn Monroe all died as a result of poisoning. Toxicology,
the study of poisons, incorporates diverse disciplines including chemistry,
biology, and botany. Patients may be poisoned accidentally or on purpose,
but either way the intensive care unit is often where they wind up. Many
poisoned patients are children or young adults, and it is especially tragic
when a young person dies in this way.

One of the deadliest poisons known to man derives from the seeds of
the castor plant. (Because of the bean-like appearance of its seed pod, it

is commonly but erroneously referred to as the castor "bean.") Its deadly nature comes from the seed's unpurified, extremely toxic extract: ricin. Inhaled, ingested, or injected, ricin usually results in a particularly gruesome death within a matter of days. It is possible to die simply by ingesting several castor beans, but death is unusual even with accidental or deliberate ingestion, because the seed's shell must be chewed or broken to expose the victim to the poison. And the plant and its seeds do have a number of uses, primarily as a form of jewelry and a household decoration. In regions of the world like India where castor plants are endemic, people are aware of the lethal nature of the castor bean and take appropriate care. It's amazing how such a deadly poison can be ubiquitous in an area and yet so few people are harmed by it—just as in the Arctic regions few people die of exposure.

The American public did not know much about ricin until it made headlines this past decade: letters laced with the poison were sent to President Obama and New York City's then-mayor, Michael Bloomberg. But what really boosted its notoriety was the immensely popular cable television show *Breaking Bad*, in which the show's protagonist, chemistry teacher turned drug kingpin Walter White, played by Bryan Cranston, used a powdered form of ricin to dispatch his enemies.

The strangest incident of ricin poisoning took place in London in 1978. Georgi Markov, a Bulgarian dissident living in political exile in Great Britain and working as a BBC broadcaster, was waiting for a bus on Waterloo Bridge. His opposition to the Communist government of Bulgaria had made him the target of several previous assassination attempts, but on that particular rainy day he perceived no special danger. During his daily midmorning commute, an unknown man appeared out of the crowd and "accidentally" poked Markov in the leg with an umbrella, causing a minor, superficial wound. Markov continued his business, thinking nothing of it.

But the incident was no accident, and it was no minor wound. Within days, Markov was dead. After a forensic investigation, ricin was recovered from his body. The man who had jabbed him was an assassin from the Bulgarian Secret Services who had been provided with a specially rigged umbrella. After the umbrella pierced Markov's skin, it implanted in the wound a pellet designed to melt at body temperature. Once the pellet decomposed, it released a dose of ricin into Markov's system—a tiny amount, but enough to kill him. At the time, there were suspicions the special umbrella and the ricin delivery system were supplied by the Russian KGB, a fact the head of the KGB actually confirmed a few years after the fact. (The pellet and a replica umbrella are now on display at "the Black Museum" at Metropolitan Police Headquarters, New Scotland Yard, London, although the exhibit is not open to the public.)

Two years later in faraway Cleveland, this international incident would have personal repercussions for me and for an unfortunate woman from central Ohio. It was my first encounter with ricin, one of the first known cases ever in the United States.

In 1980, I was working as the medical postgraduate fellow in the intensive care unit at Lakeside Hospital, part of the University Hospitals of Cleveland. This unit handled all the serious toxicology referrals for northern and central Ohio. On an August morning, the unit received a call that a woman from a rural part of the state had attempted to kill herself by ingesting castor seeds after a fight with her husband. She had been taken to a central Ohio hospital and was experiencing signs and symptoms of ricin poisoning. Now she was being airlifted to our ICU to be treated by our toxicology team. There was a problem, though: no one on the team knew anything about how to treat ricin poisoning, and since there was very little experience with ricin in North America, there was not much about it in the available medical literature.

When the young woman arrived she was quite ill and was admitted directly to the ICU. After we did our immediate evaluation, we left the room for a few minutes so the nurses could perform their duties: positioning the patient, securing the intravenous lines, attaching monitors, and recording medications. During this process, which usually takes about twenty minutes, the doctors on the medical team went to the cafeteria to discuss the case and formulate our treatment plan. One of the medical residents asked point-blank to no one in particular, "Does anyone know anything about ricin?"

There was an uncomfortable silence while we all stared at our coffee cups. We were flying blind. At that moment, I recalled the case of the Bulgarian defector.

I asked the group, "Do any of you guys know the story of that Bulgarian dissident who was stabbed with the ricin umbrella in London a couple of years ago?" More uncomfortable silence. I recounted the story of Georgi Markov, and while I was telling it, something dawned on me. "Wait a minute. You know what this means? Who knows about ricin?" Blank stares from everyone; they didn't understand where I was going. "The KGB knows about ricin poisoning!"

One of the residents launched a sarcastic riposte. "So what should we do? Call the KGB? Let me see if their Midwestern bureau number is in the telephone book."

"But don't you see? If the KGB knows about ricin, *who else* knows about ricin?"

One resident's eyes lit up because he realized what I was getting at: "*The CIA!*"

"Exactly. We can call the CIA and ask them about ricin. We may not have the KGB's number but I bet we can get a number for the CIA."

We ran this idea by the senior attending physician, who was quite a smart guy but who had a penchant for self-promotion. There are more than a few of those types in medicine, since the occasional television appearance is one of the perks of the medical profession. Our senior attending was the "TV doctor" for one of the local television stations, a role he not only took quite seriously but relished as well. The standing joke in the ICU was that the most dangerous place in Cleveland was to be caught between him and a television camera. Not surprisingly, he thought calling the CIA a great idea, more so than I realized at the time. He took control of the situation and called the medical division of the CIA in Langley, Virginia.

The doctors at Langley there took a special interest in the case. It was apparently the first publicly reported medical case involving ricin in the free world; Markov's illness was not known to be caused by ricin poisoning until the autopsy. I suspected that ricin had been used before in espionage and the military, but assumed that those reports were not available to us. The CIA medical team kept in close contact with us, and to provide advice they also connected us with scientists familiar with the poison from research centers all over the world.

The young woman who fought with her husband and swallowed castor "beans" was big news in Cleveland. It was the lead story in the evening news, and the next day's *Cleveland Plain Dealer* featured it on the front page under the headline CIA JOINS FIGHT FOR LIFE OF VICTIM OF POISON BEANS:

> A woman here who tried to kill herself is the focus of efforts by doctors at Lakeside Hospital, the Central Intelligence Agency, and international experts, all of whom are trying to keep her alive. The expertise of such a far-reaching mix of doctors was drawn together by one who remembered that the poison the woman took also was used in the celebrated assassination of Bulgarian defector Georgi I. Markov in London in 1978....
> If she does live, she may be the first known survivor of ricin poisoning. Doctors around the world will learn from her case how to diagnose other ricin poisonings.

The allusion to the doctor who remembered the Markov incident was referring not to me but to our attending physician, the TV doctor. He had a front-page picture taken at the bedside with the patient, and another one sitting in front of his bookcase looking scholarly.

To treat the patient, we performed some sophisticated washout techniques on her blood (sophisticated for 1980; today they would be considered routine). She survived, though it's quite possible she would have survived anyway. We'll never know.

I'm no different from most people: I would've liked to have gotten some credit for thinking to call the CIA. Even a brief mention would have been nice, especially since I was young and it was early in my career. But the woman lived, she and her husband were grateful, the attending physician got the credit, and the hospital got its publicity (a particular boon considering that Lakeside was in a constant publicity war with the nearby Cleveland Clinic). On the whole, everything turned out well, but it was at least in some part because of that deadly KGB umbrella.

———————

Two years later, I was the head attending physician at the University of Illinois ICU and my toxicology background from Cleveland came in handy. The ICU resident called me on a Saturday night describing a patient who had just been admitted in a coma. The resident was uncertain what was wrong, and asked if I would come right over and see the patient.

A half hour later in the ICU, I was evaluating the patient, a middle-aged biochemist at the university. Earlier that evening he had attempted suicide by ingesting something in the laboratory. The problem was that we didn't know what he had taken. I asked the police to investigate the laboratory but they found nothing suggestive there. Meanwhile, I called in the ICU pharmacologist, who always consulted on serious toxicology problems. He had never been summoned to the ICU on a Saturday night before.

When the patient was admitted to the ICU, he was near death. He was comatose, his blood pressure was extremely low, his blood was measured as very acidotic, and his skin was a mottled shade of blue. He had no more than an hour to live unless we figured out what to do.

Every hospital has available a routine toxicology analysis, which screens for common drugs but not for uncommon ones. Since we had no idea what the patient took, there was no guarantee that a routine analysis would identify what was in his blood. A biochemist would have access to an entire laboratory of poisons, so anything was possible. I had a rule for these situations:

when an unknown poison is involved, always draw extra tubes of blood and refrigerate them. At some point later on, when more information is available, those tubes may come in handy.

Based on the presentation, there were two likely possibilities for what he took, both suggested by the extreme acidity of his blood. The first possibility was a toxic alcohol derivative, like ethylene glycol. He presented in a similar manner to alcoholics who tried to drink ethylene glycol in the form of automobile antifreeze. It is extremely toxic, and the only hope of saving the patient is to put him on dialysis immediately to remove the poison. If he had taken ethylene glycol, it would show up in the sample we sent to the lab, but the sample would not be ready for at least two hours. There was no time to wait for the results, so we started dialysis immediately.

But there was another possibility, suggested by the bluish tinge to his skin, along with the acid in his blood. He may have ingested cyanide. There was, in fact, some literature to indicate that cyanide is the poison of choice among biochemists. If he had tried to commit suicide by taking cyanide, it was quite remarkable that he made it to the ICU alive. He could die at any moment.

Cyanide is classically the pill that spies in espionage thrillers carry to swallow if they are captured. In real life, it's what Nazi leaders actually used to commit suicide quickly and with certainty before they were captured. With the Russians closing in at the end of World War II, both Adolf Hitler and Josef Goebbels died instantly after taking cyanide capsules. Hitler's mistress Eva Braun also took a cyanide capsule, and Goebbels gave cyanide to his wife and six children. When the Nuremberg trials were completed, Hermann Goering, the second-highest-ranking Nazi after Hitler, was sentenced to death by hanging. He managed to cheat the hangman by secreting a cyanide capsule in his jail cell and taking it the morning he was to be hanged.

We had no time to gamble on what the patient took, and a wrong guess could be fatal. There was an antidote for cyanide. For it to be effective, it had to be administered immediately, before any tests came back. So we had to treat the patient for both potential poisons before we had evidence for

either. While we prepared to dialyze the patient for ethylene glycol ingestion, we also administered the cyanide antidote, still unsure of whether he
had ingested either of those poisons or something else entirely.

Moreover, cyanide would not be detected by the routine hospital testing
in our lab. But the pharmacologist was brilliant; he located a laboratory
that would run a cyanide test immediately on a Saturday at midnight!
Unfortunately the lab was an hour drive from the hospital. I gave the junior
intern the rest of the night off—provided he would drive to the lab and
deliver the blood sample.

Within a few minutes of sending the intern off with the sample, the
patient started improving. He was moving further from death. Was it the
cyanide antidote, the dialysis for ethylene glycol, or another poison leaving
his system? Two hours later, we had our answer. The hospital lab sample
was negative for ethylene glycol. The intern called us from the private lab
(good man—he didn't go home but waited around for the result at the lab;
that would earn him a top recommendation). It was positive for cyanide.
It appeared we had caught the patient just in time. We were lucky; so was
he. The next morning, the patient woke up. He survived without any ill
effects. It was a minor miracle.

There are a couple of postscripts to the story. To help us with dialysis,
we had called in the nephrologists. They had expected ethylene glycol,
but when that test was negative and they found out the patient had taken
cyanide, they were fascinated. This was the first time anyone had ever been
dialyzed following a cyanide overdose. Most patients who took cyanide
to kill themselves were successful before anyone reached them. For those
who ingested cyanide and actually survived to make it to the hospital, the
treatment was the cyanide antidote, not dialysis.

Of course we hadn't meant to use dialysis for a cyanide overdose. It
just happened because we were doing everything we could. Since we didn't
know that the biochemist had taken cyanide when we started dialysis, we had
provided the nephrologists with a once-in-a-lifetime opportunity. The antidote would block the effects of cyanide and save the patient's life, but in

the meantime the nephrologists had their first-ever chance to see how much cyanide was being removed from the body by dialysis. They could measure how much cyanide remained in the patient's blood and how much was in the dialysis fluid. They would have liked a cyanide level from the patient's blood before dialysis started to see how high it was and how fast they were removing it. But the sample we sent to the peripheral lab was only enough to determine whether there was cyanide in the blood, not how much of it was there. They were disappointed until I reminded them I had extra samples drawn when the patient was first brought in. That meant they could use those predialysis samples to see how high the cyanide level had been. Chances like that don't come very often.

The nephrologists collected all their information and published the first account of how dialysis would remove cyanide in a major medical journal. Thirty years later, it remains a widely cited article in both nephrology and toxicology textbooks. Shades of Cleveland: no one on my staff got any credit in the article—not even in the perfunctory "thank you" section. My residents and the pharmacologist were upset; they were right that it was unfair, and all I could do was mollify them with my story of ricin and the *Cleveland Plain Dealer*.

The second postscript was an amazing coincidence. Twenty-five years later at our Thanksgiving dinner, my cousin's father-in-law, a renowned biochemist from Northwestern, offhandedly mentioned the suicidal biochemist's name, which I happened to remember. I was stunned. It turned out they were both from Eastern Europe and had migrated to America after the war. The two biochemists had been friends in prewar Europe and had maintained their friendship in the United States ever since. My cousin's father-in-law knew of his friend's long-ago suicide attempt and brush with death, but he never realized I was the one who had taken care of him. He, too, was stunned. Over turkey that night, I told him the whole story.

I had always wondered what became of the suicidal biochemist, since patients who attempt suicide have a significant chance of repeating successfully. It turned out my worries were unfounded. The biochemist had retired soon after his suicide attempt. He apparently got a new, young girlfriend and became something of a bon vivant well into his seventies. Every year at Thanksgiving, I got an update on his activities, which apparently included frequent European ski trips. The suicidal biochemist, who had been minutes from death back in 1982, lived well into the twenty-first century, and died happily in his eighties.

10

THE WOMAN WITH THE SORE THUMB: WHY LISTENING IS AN ART

"A wise man will hear, and will increase learning,
and a man of understanding shall attain unto wise counsels."

—Proverbs 1:5

"TAKING A HISTORY" is a doctor's first encounter with a patient; it begins when the doctor asks the patient what's wrong. It's one of the first things taught in medical school, even before the physical examination of the patient. But while every student learns how to take a history, there is an art to it that is not quickly mastered. Beyond just asking the right questions, it's making eye contact with the patient, listening carefully to his or her answers, and making decisions on what to believe, what not to believe, and what to follow up on. It's akin to what lawyers do during cross-examination or what police do during interrogations. The first rule of medicine is *listen to the patients—that doesn't mean you always believe them, but you must listen to them.*

One of the pernicious trends in medical history-taking is the computer. It may have helped in many other ways, but it has not been a positive development for discussion with patients. Lawyers and police don't use computers while asking questions, and I think using computers has been detrimental for young doctors taking histories. First, fixated on the computer screen, the physician does not make eye contact with the patient. Second, one of the downsides of electronic medical records is that many of the templates are formulaic, and the doctor hesitates to deviate from computerized scripts. Nuance is lost, and important follow-up questions may not be asked. Finally, there is the practice of "cut and paste," by which the doctors simply take the information someone else has already entered. Cut and paste is a primary cause of perpetuating mistaken diagnoses and misinformation in the medical record. The first domestic case of the Ebola virus in the United States was initially misdiagnosed because of confusion in the medical record about the patient's travel history.

The computer does not acknowledge that no two patient histories are ever the same. Every patient has a different story. Then on top of that, the person taking the history must account for language and cultural differences. One of my favorite histories was when an old Southern gentleman came in one afternoon while I was working in the emergency room.

"Mr. Foster, what brought you to the hospital?"

"A Ford."

"No, I mean what was bothering you that made you come to the hospital?"

"You're the doctor. You are supposed to tell me. If I knew what was wrong, I wouldn't have come."

At this point, I realized getting this history was going to be more challenging than most. When in doubt, my rule was to ask about pain, since this is the most common complaint.

"Mr. Foster, do you have any pain?"

"I sure do."

Mr. Foster wasn't going to make it easy by telling me any more than he had to.

"Where is your pain?"

"All over."

"Can you show me where it's the worst?"

He waved his hand over his whole body, providing no additional information.

"How long have you had this pain?"

"A long time."

"Could you say how long?"

"Ever since I came from Mississippi."

"When was that?

"I told you. A long time ago."

It was time for a different approach. Sometimes the patient will divulge something when asked about their past medical history.

"Do you have any diseases?

"I sure do"

"What are they?"

"I have high blood."

"OK, what else?"

"I have low blood."

"Anything else about your blood?"

"The doctor once told me I had bad blood, but I got a shot of penicillin for that."

The layperson might wonder how someone could have "high blood" and "low blood" at the same time. Actually, not that unusual. "High blood" is a term for high blood pressure, a.k.a. hypertension. "Low blood" is a term for anemia, a low red blood cell count; it has nothing to do with hypertension, and the two can coexist. "Bad blood' is an old term for syphilis, and Mr. Foster received penicillin, the standard treatment.

"How about other diseases?"

"The doctor also told me I have sugar." Sugar is how some patients refer to diabetes.

"Any other diseases?"

"Sometimes, I fall out." That means he has intermittent seizures.

Since alcohol is such a common problem, asking about the patient's drinking history is a standard question: "Do you drink?"

"Doc, everyone drinks."

"How much do you drink?'

"Sometimes a lot, sometimes a little."

Since most alcoholics would take more care to minimize how much they drink, I doubted Mr. Foster was an alcoholic, and I abandoned that approach. But I still didn't have a clear picture of what Mr. Foster's problem was. The next step was his medication history.

"Do you take any medicines?"

Bingo.

In every patient's history there is one key question, the question critical to opening up the door to the patient's evaluation. Usually it is the first question: "What's wrong?" or "What brought you to the hospital?" Sometimes it's not the first question but the fourth or fifth. Sometimes you never ask the right question—and then you are less likely to figure out what's wrong. If a patient has an occupational disease and you never ask what kind of work she does, it is unlikely you will diagnose her correctly. If the patient contracts an infection like Lyme disease on vacation, you have to ask if he has traveled anywhere recently or you may not suspect Lyme disease.

With Mr. Foster, question #17 was the one that hit the jackpot. When I asked about his medications, he pulled out a Crown Royal bag loaded with pill bottles. Some were expired; some were duplicates. There must have been at least thirty bottles of pills prescribed by at least ten different physicians. And at the bottom of the bag was a small piece of paper. It was a discharge summary from a hospital admission a month ago. This was the Rosetta stone for Mr. Foster's case.

With the information on this piece of paper, Mr. Foster's condition became much clearer. Sometimes it just takes a little longer to get the right history. Unfortunately, today it might not happen that way. Most patients are no longer sent home with an individualized account of their hospitalization. Instead of a unique summary, the discharge paper today is a preprinted generic form that tells the patient very little and the doctor even less.

Sometimes, listening is hard.

You always want to listen to the patient and get a good history, but it's not always easy. If things are really busy, you might take shortcuts. Conversely, when things are very slow, you may not be in the right mind-set for taking a good history. Just lazy. That happened to me one night in the emergency room, and the patient taught me a valuable lesson.

I always enjoyed working in the emergency room on the overnight shift. Compared to days, the vibe was different and more my style—less administrative hassle and greater staff bonhomie, and the people working nights tended to be like-minded in their approach to taking care of patients. At County Hospital, the day shift was rap music, the evening shift was easy listening, and the overnight shift was jazz.

This time it was a slow, lazy winter night. Before midnight, we had two serious patients present within half an hour, both with severe diabetic coma. That was one of those coincidences that popped up every once in a while, the type of thing that made the emergency room interesting. After both patients were stabilized and sent to the admitting ward, we sat around for several hours with nothing to do. The waiting room was completely empty. There may have been some doctor/nurse pairing off—the stuff you see on television, but I never saw any of it and certainly never participated in any of it. (The sexy, nubile nurses didn't work that shift; they kept their date nights open.) Bored, I sat in the main trauma room reading medical journals and listening to the overnight disc jockeys on the radio.

It was about 4 AM when the nurses informed me a patient had come in, but they said it was not an emergency. The nurses were quite reliable with that type of judgment and I figured there was no hurry, so I stopped to get a cup of vending machine coffee before evaluating her.

She was an elderly black woman, in her late seventies, in no distress. She sat calmly in the examining room, waiting for a doctor, when I walked in. I looked her over, took her vitals, and concurred with the nursing assessment that it was not an emergency—the kind of case they never talk about on shows like *ER*. I wasn't mentally prepared to take a history.

"Mrs. Washington, what brought you to the hospital?"

"My thumb hurts."

"Did you bang it or mash it?" Mash was an all-purpose term for any kind of trauma.

"No, I didn't do anything to it. It just hurts."

Before I took any more history or found out anything else about her, I looked at her thumb. On gross inspection, it looked OK. I was taken aback. Why would someone come in to the emergency room at four in the morning with a sore thumb? I decided to ask her.

"Mrs. Washington, I don't understand. Why did you come to the emergency room at 4 AM with pain in your thumb?"

She immediately took the question as an affront. "Listen, *sonny* . . ." She paused for dramatic effect. "I'll tell you why I came at four in the morning. Because if I came at four in the afternoon, that waiting room would be full and I would have to sit and wait. And then you wouldn't see me until it was four in the morning. So I just decided to come at four in the morning because I knew I wouldn't have to wait. *That's why.*"

There was no denying she was right. Had she come at four in the afternoon, she would be put at the back of the line and would most likely be shunted off for twelve hours. Why not just come in at 4 AM and not have to wait?

Because I wasn't prepared to take a history, I had asked a question that offended her. To this patient, her sore thumb was as important as any other patient's problem. I made a mental note never to be so presumptuous with a patient again.

Duly chastened, I sat back, relaxed, and took a sip of coffee.

"Mrs. Washington. I have all night. I want you to tell me all about your thumb. Take your time, and tell me if there is anything else bothering you."

Her demeanor sweetened and she opened up. For the next two hours I evaluated her thumb and whatever else she wanted to talk about. She told me all about her health problems, her family, and her pets. Maybe she just came to the emergency room to talk in the first place. Some people do that. By 7 AM, the sun was coming up and I discharged her as my shift ended. She was satisfied and so was I.

As we were leaving, one of the younger residents walked out the door with me. He said, "You spent over two hours with the old lady with the thumb. Why did you spend so much time with her?" To him, Mrs. Washington was "the old lady with the thumb." It's not unusual for doctors to refer to patients by their presenting problems. Depersonalizing, but unfortunately it happens.

I said, "It's a long story. I'll tell you about it when we have some time."

———————

In the intensive care unit, people who cannot breathe for any reason frequently have breathing tubes placed in their throats. The technical term is "intubation." The tube goes through the larynx into the lungs, and it renders the patient unable to speak. When possible, the patient communicates by writing notes or by computer. It doesn't always work, but over time, ICU nurses become skilled at deciphering what intubated patients are trying to say.

Most patients are intubated for a short time, so they are incommunicado only briefly. But for those who have a breathing tube for days or even weeks, their inability to talk becomes a source of psychological strain. This frequently occurs in old people with chronic obstructive pulmonary disease (COPD). Often these patients are long-term smokers with emphysema. Years ago it wasn't unusual to see someone who had smoked two packs of cigarettes per day for fifty years, a "hundred-pack-year history" in medical vernacular. There are fewer patients like that today, although some are still around.

A doctor has to be present when the breathing tube is removed from the throat. Just as a matter of interest, I always tried to be there to hear the patient's first words after having a breathing tube removed. Think about it: you are very sick, essentially trapped in bed, in pain, uncomfortable, and unable to communicate for days. What would be your first words when you are able to speak?

Most patients don't say much when the tube is first taken out, because they are concentrating on breathing and they typically cough. They must have their mouths and throats suctioned to clear out mucus, and the best they can do at first is to muster some unintelligible grunts or some hoarse syllables. It takes them a couple of hours to reorient and gain the strength to begin talking again.

Not the longtime smokers with emphysema, though. Anyone in the ICU who has ever taken care of them knows that the minute that tube comes out, they virtually all have the same first words. It's predictable. They mount every bit of strength they have, look at you plaintively, and say in as clear a voice as possible, "I want a cigarette."

Cigarettes are what put them in the ICU in the first place, but these patients have been denied so long, and they ask so earnestly and with such conviction, that you almost feel like complying with their request. Listening to someone with emphysema after the breathing tube has been removed teaches you a lot about the grip of nicotine addiction.

11

DON'T BELIEVE EVERYTHING YOU
READ IN THE MEDICAL RECORD

"To be born with a sense of the comic is a precious heritage."

—Sir William Osler

MEDICINE IS NOW a far different profession than it was forty years ago, when I began practicing. Today, from the moment a patient enters the hospital, there are many more rules to be followed. The rules start when the patient is given his or her initial, or admitting, diagnosis. Back in the day, the admitting diagnosis was only a basic suggestion of the possibilities of what was wrong with the patient. It was left to the subsequent physicians on the ward to determine what was wrong and what should be done. Whether the admitting diagnosis was correct or not, it ceased to have implications once the patient was actually in the hospital.

The admitting diagnosis has since taken on a much greater significance for both the patient and the providers. For hospitals, private insurers, and the government, it is absolutely crucial to reimbursement, which is the sine qua non for a hospital stay. In contrast to years ago, the admitting diagnosis may bias how subsequent physicians evaluate the patient. The dilemma is explained by Dr. Robert Centor, one of the nation's leading academic internists, from the University of Alabama at Birmingham. He voiced his displeasure at the current state of affairs in his Internet blog, *db's Medical Rants*:

> Many regulations from Centers for Medicare and Medicaid Services and other insurers have influenced policies that increase anchoring and diagnostic inertia.
>
> When the emergency department physicians admit to the hospital, they have to give an admission diagnosis . . . they cannot admit for abnormal chest X-ray, or fever, but rather they must postulate a diagnosis. That diagnosis then drives case managers and protocols. Patients often receive their first treatments before the admitting physician has even met them. The emergency physicians are criticized if they do not proceed in a timely fashion. The hospital worries that they have a diagnosis that supports admission rather than observation status. If they designate the wrong status, they face a financial problem.
>
> But patients do not always arrive with diagnoses. Some diagnoses take time. Patients would benefit if the diagnosis purposely included unknown disease with manifestations rather than a diagnosis chosen for billing and quality purposes.
>
> Too often, a diagnosis induces a therapeutic freight train. And then if the patient is not discharged promptly (according to the expectations of the admission diagnosis) the admitting physician is criticized.
>
> Something is wrong with the system. (Actually much is wrong because we do not really have a system, rather we have rules.) We need ways to more acceptably label a patient as a diagnostic puzzle . . . We must develop systems to avoid diagnostic anchoring and inertia. Our patients deserve our full diagnostic attention. Unfortunately, we see too many diagnostic misadventures.

The obsession with the admitting diagnosis is one cause of medical overtesting. Here is an example of an actual case with the type of diagnostic misadventure Dr. Centor alludes to: a twenty-seven-year-old man presented to the hospital with chest pain and an abnormal ECG. The emergency physician immediately gave him an admitting diagnosis of possible myocardial infarction (heart attack). This diagnosis automatically sets off a chain reaction of people summoned to the hospital, including a cardiologist to do an immediate cardiac catheterization—a test that involves injecting dye into the vessels that supply the heart.

When the team assembled, the cardiologist arrived last, evaluated the patient, and determined the chest pain was unlikely related to the heart. The cardiologist read the ECG and realized it was simply a variant of a normal ECG—i.e., not a problem. He knew the young man was not having a heart attack. *But he did the catheterization anyway*, because the rules required it based on the admitting diagnosis. Not to do the catheterization would be bad for the hospital metrics for chest pain treatment (how long it takes for a patient with chest pain to have a cardiac catheterization), which could ultimately harm reimbursement status. Thousands of dollars later and with some risk attached to the procedure, the young man's catheterization results were normal.

Years ago when I worked in the emergency room, the admitting diagnosis wasn't crucial for payment, and admitting doctors used it only as an initial guide to evaluating the patient. As Dr. Centor noted, determining the correct diagnosis can take time.

———

At urban hospitals like Cook County, the emergency room saw a large number of patients who were admitted to the hospital for social rather than medical reasons: old people who could no longer take care of themselves; alcoholics who had no place to go for shelter; poor people who were the victims of various types of abuse and neglect. Technically, most of these people did not have a medical diagnosis, but they had to be admitted to the hospital nevertheless. The admitting diagnosis wasn't really important. This was the hospital at the crossroads of medicine and social service.

These patients tended to come to the emergency room in the middle of the night. Every evening, there were old people and homeless people just lying on stretchers for hours waiting to go to the admitting ward. Often the junior residents would ask me what admitting diagnosis to put in for these people so they could be admitted for social reasons. At first, I took the conventional approach. I told them to write down pneumonia, heart failure, or some other common diagnosis. But I soon noticed that once these patients were admitted, they often got tests and treatments they didn't need, because they didn't really have those conditions. They needed social services, not a lot of tests. Once in a while something bad happened to them because of unnecessary testing.

Seeing that, I tried a new, more lighthearted approach to the admitting diagnosis. No one was monitoring what admitting diagnosis was entered, so I had the emergency room residents put in things like "social service deficiency" or "hyperacute domiciliary shortage." My favorite for the elderly was "failure to thrive." This is a legitimate diagnosis for sick newborns, meaning that for some reason they are not gaining weight at the appropriate rate. (Ironically, today it has also become an acceptable admitting diagnosis for old people who are just not doing well.)

This novel, nonmedical approach to admitting diagnoses met with some disfavor among some of the admitting doctors on the wards. Those with a sense of humor understood what I was doing and had no problem going along. Another group did not see the humor and made a point of letting me know that "every patient must have a legitimate admitting medical diagnosis." More likely than not, those doctors were the ones who had sat in the front row of class in medical school and scored highest on the multiple choice tests. Humorless.

But since those doctors wanted an admitting diagnosis, they would get one. I began checking the list of patients to be admitted, and which doctors they would be admitted to. For patients admitted from the emergency room for purely social reasons, I would choose a rare medical diagnosis that had nothing to do with the patient's condition. And to make sure the doctors didn't take the diagnoses too literally and start doing a bunch of tests, I selected obscure, exotic tropical diseases like "chronic indolent trypanosomiasis" (sleeping sickness), "acute Ross River Fever" (a viral infection caused by mosquitos in Papua, New Guinea) or, "possible subacute loa-loa" (a disease caused by an equatorial roundworm). Imagine seeing the face of the doctor who received a ninety-year-old patient from the emergency room with an admitting diagnosis of equatorial roundworm. But the fake diagnoses did the trick: the patients were admitted and not subjected to potentially harmful testing or procedures.

Eventually, of course, I was reprimanded by my superiors for this unorthodox approach and I was forced to revert to the conventional system. But if those thirty-five-year-old County charts and their admitting diagnoses could be reviewed today, the reviewer would no doubt wonder about the unexplained outbreak of rare tropical diseases among geriatric patients in Chicago.

———————————

One evening, these fictional admitting diagnoses in emergency room patients had an unexpectedly humorous result. An old alcoholic came in, medically stable, but he was one of those patients who had to be admitted for detoxification so that social services could find a place for him to stay.

Before he was admitted, even though he had no breathing problems, I obtained a chest X-ray, because some such patients carried tuberculosis. The X-ray surprised everyone in the emergency room—it revealed that his left lung was completely nonfunctional because it was calcified, most likely as a result of old, burned-out tuberculosis or perhaps an occupational lung disease—say, from long-ago work as a coal miner. It was obviously a chronic condition and had no clinical significance at this time, but it was a striking chest X-ray.

The X-ray was up in the emergency room view box when one of the surgeons walked by. He stopped in his tracks and, like everyone else, was taken aback by the startling picture.

"Whoa, what is *that*?"

I explained to him that it was pulmonary calcification from some past disease but it wasn't germane to his current medical problems. The medical term was "an incidental finding." The surgeon, obviously impressed by the X-ray, asked me, "Does that condition have a name?"

It didn't. But the surgeon's name was Dr. Earle and I said to him, "Well, it will now. We're going to name this calcified lung condition after you. It's now known as Earle's lung. It's the first case—you just became famous. How many people get a disease named after them?"

"Right. Even if it's not really a disease. Besides, it's the first case—and the only case," he replied.

"Most likely the only case any of us will ever see," I added.

After that, the patient had to be admitted to the hospital and I needed an admitting diagnosis. This time, the diagnosis would be obvious: Earle's lung. Of course, there was no such thing and no one had ever heard of it, but there it was on the X-ray.

Not surprisingly, the X-ray was the talk of the next morning's conference even though the patient's condition had nothing to do with his lung. Earle's lung? What was that? I came to morning report and told everyone Earle's lung was a rare calcific condition of the lung. Everyone bought the fictional diagnosis.

Fortunately for my case of Earle's lung, there was no Internet; no one could Google the term and find there was no match. One resident did mention that he looked Earle's lung up in his textbook and couldn't find it, which he thought was strange. I told him that it was a rare condition and he would probably have to consult an older textbook in the library. He believed it.

I did not anticipate the epilogue to the story. The patient was on the ward, doing well. His medical record diagnoses were alcoholism and Earle's lung. Even after several days, still no one had figured out that Earle's lung was a fake diagnosis. Perhaps someone even hypothesized a clinical connection between alcoholics and Earle's lung.

But about a week into his hospitalization on the ward, the patient suffered a severe allergic medication reaction. His blood pressure dropped very low, and he had to be transferred to the ICU. I learned what happened there from an ICU resident.

His superior, the ICU attending, was a pulmonary physician and the resident presented the case to her when the patient was transferred to the ICU: "Patient is a fifty-nine-year-old male with a history of Earle's lung, who suffered an allergic reaction on the ward . . ."

After the resident finished the presentation, the ICU attending examined the patient and gathered everyone to the ICU X-ray view box, where they all saw the amazing X-ray. The residents were curious to see the attending physician's reaction, hoping to learn about this rare lung disease.

She was reassuring. "It's rare, but I've seen several cases of Earle's lung." Interesting, but of course impossible, because there was no such disease.

———————

Decades before, my father had pulled a similar trick on the doctors. In the early 1950s, as one of the chief physicians at County, he worked with the pathologists there. Several of these pathologists were world renowned, having emigrated from prestigious European universities before World War II to Chicago, when it was a center of American medicine. They held a conference where pathologists from across the Midwest would come and examine clinical slides prepared from patients' biopsy specimens.

There were famous pathologists, some with large egos, attending those conferences. Everyone wanted to be the one who guessed the clinical condition from the slides, which my father was responsible for preparing. One day, in preparing the slides, unbeknownst to anyone, he took a piece of delicatessen salami, did the tissue stains, and presented that instead of a patient's biopsy specimen. None of these pathologists had a clue what the tissue was; they guessed all sorts of diseases from every organ in the body. It remained an unknown, and ultimately some of the country's best pathologists were stumped by a piece of sandwich meat.

12

SOURCES OF EMBARRASSMENT: VIBRATORS, RASHES, AND MEDICAL STUDENTS

"It's an incredible paradox that being a doctor is so degrading and yet is so valued by society."

—DR. SAMUEL SHEM, *HOUSE OF GOD*

H OSPITALS HAVE BEEN the setting of so many successful melodramas and comedies on radio and then television, if for no other reason than because they are a fount of emotion. Stories of life and death make for a constant source of drama. But there are other contributors to the drama, including the rigid hospital hierarchy of attending physicians, residents, and medical students; the interplay between different specialties and how they jealously guard their turf; and of course the never-ending dynamic between doctors and nurses. The interactions of all of these dramatis personae put emotions, including love, anger, and frustration, on continual display.

Another emotion always at work is embarrassment. The hospital can be an embarrassing place, and not just for patients who have to wear those gowns that expose their backsides.

Take the case of the nurse and the vibrator. At some point, almost every emergency room has seen the phenomenon of rectal foreign bodies. Most commonly, patients have inserted objects in their rectums for sexual gratification. But there are other reasons as well. Criminals will occasionally conceal drug packets or weapons rectally. Psychiatric patients have been known to conceal sharp objects in their rectums to harm those they believe are threatening them. And some patients simply swallow foreign bodies, which go through the gastrointestinal tract and wind up stuck in the rectum.

The list of objects that doctors have extracted from rectal cavities is long and frankly amazing. It has, on occasion, included live animals. Sometimes the doctors must remove more than one object, generally after the embarrassed patient inserted a second object in an unsuccessful attempt to extract the first. The diagnosis is usually not difficult, as most patients will confess why they came to the hospital, although they often concoct implausible stories about having sat on the offending object. As part of the evaluation, it is mandatory to obtain X-rays of the object(s) in the rectum; there is an ample array of such pictures to browse on the Internet as confirmation, for anyone so inclined.

With the right equipment, most foreign bodies can be removed in the emergency room, but when an article is breakable—for example, a light bulb—the patient may have to be taken to the operating room for extraction. Likewise, if the object has migrated farther up the rectum into the colon, it may be impossible to remove unless the patient is sent to the operating room for general anesthesia.

Among the most frequently encountered articles are vibrators. I saw one case in which the vibrator had traveled so high into the rectum that it was impossible to remove in the emergency room. The surgeons were called to take the patient to the operating room, where the patient could be anesthetized and it was possible to visualize the vibrator directly. In the operating room, the surgeons inserted a scope to locate the object's exact position and then slipped a snare past the vibrator. They captured it and gradually nudged it down the colon, into the rectum, and finally outside the body.

At that point, the vibrator became a surgical specimen, and it was treated like any other object or tissue removed from the body. The surgeon called for a specimen tray and the nurses brought one to the table. All fairly routine.

Except that as the doctors placed the vibrator on the specimen table with the snare, someone inadvertently hit the power switch. The vibrator was still in working order and it turned on. At that point, doctors, nurses, and an anesthesiologist saw a vibrator vibrating on the specimen table in front of them. Everyone was taken aback; they all just stood there for a moment looking on helplessly.

It was then that a circulating nurse, whose job it was to monitor all the activities in the operating theaters, happened to peer into the room. All she could see was a bunch of perplexed people just standing around. She entered the room, assessed the situation, and took charge. She put on some gloves and simply switched the vibrator off. She was obviously familiar with vibrator controls. The rest of the staff did not let the embarrassed nurse forget that for some time.

Embarrassing things happen to doctors as well. One night at the nurses' station, I was reviewing some charts. It was a quiet evening, nothing much happening, and there were three other doctors around. One was the chief medical resident, who is the ranking medical officer in the hospital at night, and another was the chief surgery resident, his surgical counterpart. I had no idea who the third resident was. He was sitting quietly in the corner, writing a note. The two chief residents were going over the charts on patients they were responsible for when the chief medical resident saw something he considered funny and turned to the chief surgery resident, "Look at this. Someone called a STAT dermatology consult."

A "STAT consult" means a patient must be seen immediately. The chief medical resident was amused that someone would call in dermatologists in the evening to see a patient right away. The chief surgical resident shared his amusement and asked rhetorically, "Who the hell calls a STAT derm consult?"

They both began laughing uncontrollably at the thought of someone considering a skin problem an emergency. At that point, the quiet resident in the corner looked up. It turned out he was the dermatology resident who had been called. He had heard the entire conversation and approached the desk where the other two sat. Feeling disrespected, he was confrontational.

"What do you mean, 'Who the hell calls a STAT derm consult?'"

He might have been joking. I wasn't sure, especially as he continued by addressing them each as "Mr." rather than "Dr.": "Hoo, hoo. Two big shots. Mr. Big Shot Medical Chief Resident. Let me tell you something. If a patient has a myocardial infarction, it will be there tomorrow morning. And Mr. Big Shot Chief Surgical Resident, if a patient has acute appendicitis, he will be there tomorrow morning. But if you don't call your derm consults STAT, *the rash might be gone in the morning.*"

The two embarrassed chiefs did not know what to say. I said nothing, smiling to myself. Of course, the dermatology resident was right.

———

When it comes to embarrassment in the hospital, no one can humiliate like a bullying, aggressive attending physician, especially if he is pitted against a timid resident who has little confidence. This time it was in July, when the new residents were assuming their duties for the first time. A shy new resident was called on to present his first case to one of the dinosaur attendings, a veteran of decades of case presentations. This dinosaur was notorious for giving newbies a hard time. Nothing good will come of this, I thought.

The resident started his presentation calmly. He discussed the patient's case, which was terminal cancer in an elderly man. When he was done presenting, the attending physician eyed him suspiciously. "Dr. Harris, how is the patient doing this morning?"

"He died last night, sir."

"He *what*?"

"He died, sir."

The attending physician exploded: "HARRIS, WE GIVE YOU AN EDUCATION. WE GIVE YOU TRAINING. WE GIVE YOU THE RESPONSIBILITY OF TAKING CARE OF OUR PATIENTS. AND AS SOON AS WE DO, WHAT DO YOU DO? YOU LET THEM DIE? IS THAT WHAT YOU DO? WHAT DO YOU HAVE TO SAY FOR YOURSELF?"

It was all an act designed to embarrass the poor resident. I saw him do that—or something close to it—a hundred times to intimidate young doctors. The patient was terminal and he knew it, so his death really wasn't an issue. The resident hadn't done anything wrong. But he turned red as the attending continued his tirade. "WELL, HARRIS? I'M WAITING. THE FIRST TIME WE GIVE YOU SOME RESPONSIBILITY AND YOU LET YOUR PATIENTS DIE? YOU CALL YOURSELF A DOCTOR? WHAT DO YOU HAVE TO SAY FOR YOURSELF?"

The embarrassed resident looked at him sheepishly and stammered, "S-S-S-S-Sir, I'm w-w-w-w-wondering if I c-c-c-c-can have an-n-n-n-nother chance."

The room grew silent. Nobody laughed out loud, but everyone smiled. Even the attending physician, who thought he'd heard everything, was suppressing a laugh. He just grinned, shook his head, and said, "OK. Next case."

———————

No one embarrasses like attending physicians, and it is a sad fact that no one endures embarrassment like medical students. They work so hard to make it into medical school, and then, for four years, they are often forced to endure all sorts of indignities. The worst embarrassment I ever saw a medical student suffer was at a Saturday morning surgical conference with the city's top surgeons. Unfortunately, I was partly to blame for the embarrassing incident.

Fifty of Chicago's best surgeons met weekly to discuss various cases and surgical techniques and exchange thoughts. Good surgeons are great doctors, but they can be merciless with underlings. In this conference, they were often brutal with their remarks and in their approach. I made it a point to attend, and to bring my residents and students. As an internist, I was an outsider, but I had learned not to be deterred by their bluster. Though I was not a surgeon, I liked to attend the conference for two reasons.

First of all, the surgeons served the best doughnuts and coffee. They rarely skimped on refreshments at conferences, and food is always a major draw for a hospital conference. If you serve lunch, you can increase attendance by 50 percent. If the food is actually good, you might double the number of attendees. The pharmaceutical industry has made billions of dollars by exploiting that simple fact.

Another reason to attend their conference was that the surgeons knew things internists didn't know, things I wanted to learn myself and teach my students. Surgeons had facts at their command I didn't possess and they approached problems differently than internists did. Sometimes their approach was better, sometimes it was worse, but either way it was instructive. As the saying goes, "Nothing is ever a complete failure; it can always serve as a bad example."

In a room filled with surgeons, being the only internist invites suspicion. They would ask questions such as "Why are you here?" or "Is this some kind of quality assurance check?" Occasionally they actually would ask, "Are you some kind of spy?" I think they were joking.

If I told them I was there to learn, it did not placate them in the least. In fact, it often made them more suspicious. I sat through conferences as the target of hostile stares. I would shrug them off, wink, and just get something else to eat. Sometimes I would tell them, "I'm here for the doughnuts."

Some of them actually did buy that answer. They believed that assertion more than they believed I just wanted to learn from them. It's just the way surgeons and internists interact sometimes.

This particular Saturday morning I brought my best resident, and a junior medical student tagged along. It would be the perfect opportunity for a young student to observe and acclimate to an intimidating environment among imperious surgeons.

This is the profession you are entering, young man. Be prepared.

We got our doughnuts and sat in the middle of the conference room. My resident, aware we were considered interlopers, asked why we were sitting in "the belly of the beast."

I told him, "If you are going in the shark tank, it's more interesting being thrown in the deep end."

The resident, with a sense of the absurd, smiled. The student was silent. He was almost white with fright. He had never been in an atmosphere like this before.

While the surgeons were filing in, I asked my resident to give me some background on the student. Apparently before medical school, he had gone to Caltech or somewhere like that, and had worked on guidance systems for intercontinental ballistic missiles.

I said, "The kid worked on ICBMs? You know that makes him the smartest guy in the room."

Once the surgeons picked up on the intruders in the auditorium, there were the obligatory glares. One surgeon asked, "What are you doing here?"

I was in a flippant mood so I told him we were spying on him. He turned to my resident and asked if he was with me. He shrugged his shoulders and laughed. The surgeons simply ignored the medical student as though his seat was empty. They looked right through him.

The conference began with the orthopedic surgeons presenting the case of a seventy-five-year-old woman who was discovered on the floor in her home. She had apparently fallen and broken her femur. As they were about to discuss the surgical management of her fracture, my resident nudged me.

"What is it?"

"The student wants to ask a question."

That was a bold move. He would be forced to stand, an alien in a hostile world. If his question was stupid, they would eat him alive.

But I gave my blessing because I just didn't think they would turn on a student who was with me. My resident did not share my confidence, but he was waiting to see what would happen. I told the student, "Go ahead. Ask away."

The student raised his hand. From the stage, the head surgeon called on him to stand up. The young man's voice cracked, and you could tell that he was scared. The surgeons in particular can smell fear. A baby antelope among the lions.

In a trembling voice the student asked, "How do you know the lady fell and broke her femur? How do you know she didn't break her femur and then fall?"

It was the old question—chicken or the egg. He said his piece and sat down very quickly.

There was a brief moment of silence. Then laughter. The surgeon at the microphone said, "That might be the stupidest question I have ever heard in this conference."

More laughter. And stares. And a couple of nasty comments from the audience. The crowd was turning on him. I hadn't anticipated a reaction this vicious. I felt bad for the student. Just when I thought it couldn't get worse, it did.

The resident leaned over to me and said, "He's crying."

"What?"

"He's crying."

I looked over and, sure enough, the student was sobbing. He was completely humiliated. And the whole room was staring at him.

My resident gave me a disapproving look. "Nice work."

I had that coming. I could have prevented this simply by telling him not to ask his question, but I thought I could protect him.

My resident asked, "Well, what do we do now?"

I said, "We have to get him out of here, right away."

I stood up and motioned them to leave. It turned out it had been a bad idea to choose seats in the middle of the room. Imagine standing up and walking through the middle aisle during the most dramatic act of a play that is completely sold out. Multiply that by one hundred and you have an idea. The three of us—me, an amused resident, and a sobbing student.

It seemed like an eternity before we got out of that conference room. I took the student outside and put my arm around him. The crying just got worse.

I said, "I'm sorry. I shouldn't have let you go in front of those guys. They're jerks."

After a minute or two, he began to regain his composure. He was still sobbing and became apologetic even though he had done nothing wrong. Through the sobs he stuttered, "I'm-I'm-I'm r-r-r-r-r-eally s-s-s-s-sorry."

I said, "You have nothing to be sorry about."

While my resident talked him down, I was trying to think of something else to console him. Suddenly, it dawned on me. The surgeons had laughed at him, and then humiliated him, but there is one thing they didn't do.

I said to him, "I just want you to remember one thing. Think about this: they never answered your question."

Perhaps he heard me, perhaps not. He left quickly and I never found out what became of him. I doubt he went into surgery.

This all happened in the time before the medical community understood much about osteoporosis and how patients can have spontaneous fractures from brittle bones. While most fractures are caused by falls, a certain percentage are caused by osteoporosis. It was certainly possible that the old lady they presented that day did indeed have a spontaneous fracture and then fell. The student's query was a classic cause-and-effect question, one of the hardest ones to answer in medicine.

My resident went on to become a prestigious attending physician in another state. He would visit when he came to Chicago and we would reminisce. One evening over dinner I asked if he remembered the medical student who had been humiliated in the surgical conference years before.

He laughed and teased me, "Sure I do. You did a real nice job protecting him from the surgeons."

Guilty as charged. But I reminded him, "No one in the room considered the possibility of a spontaneous fracture. It turned out to be a more intelligent question than you, I, or anyone else realized."

13

THE MYSTERY OF
THE SEDUCTIVE NURSE

––––––––––

"The joy of medicine is the challenge of making
a solid diagnosis, the delight in besting (if only momentarily)
an intern or resident, the satisfaction (if rare) of actually helping
someone, the sheer cantankerousness of being able to tell
the bureaucracy to 'stuff it.'"

—Dr. Michael J. Halberstam

THERE WAS NEVER a better description of making a diagnosis than this one offered by the late, renowned cardiologist Michael Halberstam (coincidentally, the brother of journalist David Halberstam). I got my first taste of that joy as a senior student, when I made a true diagnosis of something that no one else had suspected.

The patient was a pediatric intensive care nurse, but not at our hospital. She'd been off work for more than a year and had been in and out of a number of hospitals with an unknown illness. Her problem was "fever of unknown origin," medical jargon for an unexplained, intermittent rise in body temperature. In her case, the fevers would occasionally climb as high as 105°F.

Fever of unknown origin is a difficult diagnostic problem, because there are so many potential causes. It is a subject of frequent discussion in journals and books. Here is a partial list of the possible causes and their likelihood:

Causes of Fever of Unknown Origin

Infection (20–40%)

  Tuberculosis

  Infective endocarditis

  Epstein-Barr virus (EBV)

  Cytomegalovirus (CMV)

Connective tissue disorders (20%)

  Rheumatoid arthritis

  Systemic Lupus Erythematosus

  Adult-onset Still's disease

  Temporal arteritis

Malignancy (10–20%)

  Lymphoma

  Leukemia

  Hepatocellular carcinoma

Undiagnosed (20%)

Drugs (10%)

With such a wide range of potential diagnoses, the number of tests, procedures, and surgeries a patient could undergo is staggering.

For someone who had been in so many hospitals, the young woman looked remarkably healthy when she was admitted to the ICU. Not your typical chronic ICU patient. Shortly after she was admitted, she started spiking fevers and had a transient fall in her blood pressure. This suggested a bacterial infection in the blood, but why had no one diagnosed such a routine condition up until this point?

One hospital had recorded a positive blood culture of an extremely unusual organism, which might have explained the fevers, but every repeat blood culture was negative. The lack of any other positive blood cultures just added to the puzzle. Perhaps an infection wasn't the cause of her fevers. Meanwhile at every hospital, specialists of every stripe visited her constantly—infectious disease specialists, rheumatologists, oncologists, cardiologists, gastroenterologists, surgeons—each with his or her own pet theory. She had biopsies, blood tests, scans, X-rays, everything, with no answers.

Our hospital repeated the same routine; there was no reason not to. It's quite common for a patient to go from a community hospital to a university hospital, where most or all of the tests would be repeated. One problem with this approach is that it doesn't encourage new thinking about the patient as often as it should. Electronic medical records were meant to address this problem of duplicated tests, but in truth they have probably done little more than make a small dent.

After a couple of days, the hospital's best specialists held conferences about the patient's condition—with no good answers. The main theory had to do with her exposure to children as a pediatric nurse; the most likely possibility was that she must have contracted some rare infection or virus from a child. But not a single test was positive. As the student in the ICU, my role was to review all the records from the other hospitals. This entailed going through thousands of pages of records because she'd been in these hospitals for weeks at a time. Lots of tests with no answers. One thing that struck me was that *she chose to come to a different hospital every time to have the same tests over again.* That was a little strange, especially for a nurse who knew that was likely to happen. Why would she knowingly subject herself to the same tests over and over?

I raised that question with my seniors, but it didn't make an impression on them. They had their own long, detailed workup planned for her. After combing through her records, I was ready to assess her personally.

There was nothing in her history or physical exam to explain what was wrong; if there had been, someone would have seen it long before me. The only thing that was remarkable was the number of scars she had from various hospital procedures and biopsies. In addition, she'd had so many intravenous lines that her skin veins were impossible to access, so she had a large IV line placed in the vein of her neck, just like the drug addicts I would care for who destroyed their own veins.

But talking with her raised my suspicions. She was about my age, and quite attractive. Had we met in a social setting, I might have considered asking her for a date. (In a professional setting, however, that is a boundary that should not be crossed.) I found it easy to talk with her and get to know her, which I felt was crucial. *Always listen to the patient.*

She was seductive—not necessarily in a physical sense, but it was clear that she spoke in a manner that was designed to win my trust. She was alternately flattering, then helpless, then beseeching me to help her. But I thought to myself, she knew I was only the student, with little control over her care. How could I help her when the best specialists were on her case? With plenty of hospital experience and an intimate familiarity with the hospital hierarchy, she knew I couldn't.

I asked her about the workups she'd had at the other hospitals. Her mood changed immediately. She morphed from helpless young woman in the throes of illness to aggrieved medical professional. She told me these people were all idiots. Every one of those hospitals, every one of those doctors. They couldn't figure out what was wrong. They had no idea what they were doing. When I told her she would receive basically the same workup here, she told me she had confidence that we were smarter, with a better reputation. She knew we could find the problem.

To me, that seemed like disingenuous sweet talk. Another thing that didn't sit well with me was her dismissive attitude toward her nurses. She didn't like any of them. Most nurses who are hospitalized are protective of the nurses who take care of them. They understand.

Before I left the room, she asked me to make sure her intravenous line was working. Surely her nurses were doing that. Why did she ask me? I checked with her nurse, who told me it had been looked at several times already that morning. Her nurse didn't like her at all—a sure sign that something was amiss.

I also reviewed her fever chart and noticed that since she had been in the ICU, she'd had no fever spikes during the day. The only time she ran a fever was at night. That was unlike her previous hospital patterns, and it didn't jibe with most of the diseases everyone was looking for.

I had been taught by extremely smart older physicians always to keep my radar up when interviewing patients, and my limited experience had reinforced that lesson. The common mistake many doctors make is that they do only one interview with a patient. Sometimes more than one interview is necessary.

I went back to speak with her a second time, less to gain information than to sense her mood. Again, I was met with the verbal seduction. But I harbored no illusions; I knew that if I joined the ranks of those who couldn't figure this out, she would simply consider me another idiot. On a whim, I asked her if she knew that her fevers in the ICU were occurring only at night. She denied she knew that. There was no way an intensive care nurse with her history wouldn't notice a pattern like that in her own fever curve. She eyed me suspiciously and asked me, "What do you think it means?"

Parry and thrust. I countered with, "What do you think it means?"

Then she gave her first openly hostile answer to me: "*How should I know?* You're supposed to be the doctor. But you're only a student anyway."

I had been asked to leave patients' rooms before because I was only a student. Some patients don't want students taking care of them; others don't mind. It was no big deal to me to be the low rung on the ladder. Normally, I would have written off that remark as the frustrations of a sick patient who has not been treated well by the medical system. But this was too quick and too mercurial. Only minutes before I had been part of the brilliant team that would solve her problem.

I shrugged, said nothing, and left the room. Later, on the evening shift, I returned on the pretense of dropping in to say hello. She looked distressed, but her temperature was normal. I gave her the results of some of her lab values: they were all normal; she seemed completely dismissive and sent me away. It was almost as if she didn't care what was wrong with her. Her attitude was unlike that of any patient I had ever seen. That's when I had an idea. I asked one of the overnight nurse's aides to do me a favor: *Keep a special eye on that patient tonight. If you can, see what she is doing when she thinks nobody is paying attention to her.* I suspected the patient might be doing something to induce her fever at night.

During the day in the ICU it would have been hard to do that, because there were so many people around. But at night, not so hard. As a nurse, maybe she knew a special trick to manipulate the thermometers. But people watched her for that, and besides, to manipulate a thermometer to read as high as 105°F would be hard to do. Still, she was a nurse and a clever one at that.

The nurse's aide was an older woman who had been around the block. She knew what I was asking. She trusted me. More important, she didn't trust the patient.

She broke the case that the top doctors in the city couldn't break.

In the middle of the night, the patient did indeed spike a fever to 105°F. The nurse called the physician, they did the same cultures that had been done so many times before, and gradually after an hour the patient's temperature came down. Then next morning I came in early and saw that the patient had spiked a fever the night before. I planned on talking to the nurse's aide in the evening, assuming she had gone home at the end of her shift. But she hadn't. She was calmly sipping tea, waiting for me in the ward break room.

"Mrs. Daniels, how come you haven't gone home?

"I had to talk to you, Dr. Franklin." (Technically I was still a student and did not merit the title "doctor," but she did not make that distinction.)

"What is it?"

"Dr. Franklin, I saw what that girl did right before they took her temperature."

What she told me next stunned me.

"About 2 AM, she didn't think anyone was watching her, but I saw her go to her purse. She took out a syringe and a specimen cup that had a little urine in it. She took out a little urine with the syringe and injected it into the intravenous line in her neck. Then she got a shaking fever. But before the nurses got back, she hid everything."

"Did you tell anyone?"

"I thought I would tell you first."

"Thanks, Mrs. Daniels."

Most likely, Mrs. Daniels did not want to say anything because it would have been her word against the patient's, and in those days she probably figured an elderly black woman on the night shift might not win that argument in the hospital against a young white patient who also happened to be a nurse. That was probably true.

I immediately went to the attending physician. Like me, he was stunned. He confronted the patient and she initially denied everything. When the head nurse asked if she would consent to having her purse searched, she initially resisted. Then she realized that would be a tacit admission of guilt and finally agreed. Just as the aide had said, there was a small syringe, a cup of urine (it was her own), and a couple of needles. She confessed to injecting her own urine to produce fevers. She had been doing it for more than a year. She had confounded everyone and that's why all the tests were negative except for that one culture of her blood. It was probably the only time the doctors drew her blood soon enough to capture the organism that she injected into her blood from infected urine. The patient's diagnosis, the one that no hospital or specialist had made, was Munchausen syndrome. The website of the Cleveland Clinic defines it this way:

Munchausen syndrome is a type of factitious disorder, or mental illness, in which a person repeatedly acts as if he or she has a physical or mental disorder when, in truth, he or she has caused the symptoms. People with factitious disorders act this way because of an inner need to be seen as ill or injured, not to achieve a concrete benefit, such as financial gain. They are even willing to undergo painful or risky tests and operations in order to get the sympathy and special attention given to people who are truly ill. Some will secretively injure themselves to cause signs like blood in the urine or cyanosis of a limb. Munchausen syndrome is a mental illness associated with severe emotional difficulties.

Munchausen syndrome—named for Baron von Munchausen, an 18th century German officer who was known for embellishing the stories of his life and experiences—is the most severe type of factitious disorder. Most symptoms in people with Munchausen syndrome are related to physical illness—symptoms such as chest pain, stomach problems, or fever—rather than those of a mental disorder.

In the 1970s, Munchausen syndrome was not well understood. Today, it is far better researched and reported than it was then. The attending physician wrote a case report in a medical journal about the young nurse who injected herself with urine. It was one of the first descriptions of the syndrome and even today, forty years later, it remains one of the better ones.

14

THE PRINCESS AND THE KING

"Elvis is dead and I don't feel so good myself."

—Lewis Grizzard

I T WAS ABOUT a year before the infamous car accident in a Paris tunnel that shocked Great Britain and the rest of the world. At County, someone in hospital security slipped me the top-secret word: Princess Diana would be making an hour-long tour of the hospital the first week in June. News of celebrity visits to Cook County Hospital is guarded with the diligence reserved for national security clearance. Yet the whole thing quickly becomes a dead giveaway because of the cleaning and painting that starts immediately. It is reminiscent of the scene in the movie *Stalag 17* in which the Germans make the American POW barracks look like the Hilton when Red Cross inspectors visit. The next day, back to the usual.

Painters had been furiously at work in hospital stairwells that hadn't seen a fresh coat since Elvis was in short pants. Dust that had been gathering for the better part of a century was being steam cleaned off the corridors. I asked one tradesman if he knew what all this was about.

"Overtime," he replied tersely. Here was a man with his priorities straight.

Eventually, the state secret was released and the signs that royalty was visiting were obvious. Some local cynics voiced a sentiment that this princess-worship stuff was evidence of what rubes we Chicagoans are. I must confess when I first heard she was coming, I felt the same way as the skeptics. Yet I saw an opportunity for my daughters that I didn't want to miss.

Lacking that certain je ne sais quoi that would make me part of the official greeting group, I hatched my plan. The princess would have to pass by my office for access to the only stairway on her official route. If I played my cards right, I could bring my daughters (truants from school for the day) to my office. At the right instant, we would emerge for a moment of prime face time with Lady Di. It was all in the timing.

On the big day, every parking space around the hospital was cleared. One illegally situated Chevy, mocking all efforts at parking enforcement, was finally towed with an accompanying stack of parking tickets thicker than a mediocre Russian novel. Coincidentally, that day's staff medical lecture was anorexia nervosa and bulimia, and since the princess herself suffered from an eating disorder, some unsung hero had the good sense to remove the posters advertising it.

I put my plan into action and my daughters were ensconced in my office a half hour before the big moment. Finally, the princess arrived. Each time a celebrity visits, the same routine ensues at County: politicians, administrators, bureaucrats, and even some doctors who have never been seen there before are everywhere. As the princess made her rounds, the hospital was abuzz.

The security guard assigned to my stairwell was philosophical as he eyed the swelling crowds. "One man's headache is another man's joy," he opined stoically. There was something comforting in such wisdom. True to form, he was cool—when I apprised him of my plan, he motioned to my daughters to stand right in front as the princess approached. When she arrived, she cut a striking figure in her powder-blue outfit. She accepted a flower from my daughters, and graciously shook hands with both of them before moving on. Like everyone else, we were enthralled.

My plan had worked! Unfortunately, I had only a split second to decide whether to shake her hand or to hold my large camcorder and capture the moment when my kids met the princess. If you're not a father, go ask someone who is. Though I did not shake hands with Diana, I did earn some consolation that evening watching television news about the rest of her Chicago visit. Luck and a kind security guard had afforded my daughters the same privilege as those people at the Field Museum who had paid thousands of dollars for a dinner with the princess. It's something they will be able to tell their children.

That day changed my mind about the supposed frivolousness of princess-worship. Waiting to see her on that hospital corridor were County employees of disparate backgrounds, some born in Bridgeport, some born on the Mississippi Delta, some from the outskirts of Manila, Seoul, or Mexico City. None of them had the remotest connection with the British Empire or royalty. Yet the joy and enchantment on each and every face as Lady Di greeted them and shook their hands was undeniable. For days, that hour was the main topic of conversation at the hospital, even among rabid Bulls fans in the middle of the NBA Finals during the Michael Jordan era. I don't pretend to understand it, but there is something to this princess business, and it is genuine.

It turned out to be Diana's last visit to the city; any hope of her ever coming to Chicago again disappeared the next autumn in Paris.

If Elvis weren't dead, he would be in his eighties now. People no longer talk as much about him still being alive, probably because his graying fans don't want to imagine the King of Rock 'n' Roll as an octogenarian. There was a time when "Elvis approaching eighty" would conjure up visions of a hot 1957 Thunderbird, top down, Ann-Margret or some other starlet at his side with the wind blowing through her hair outside Las Vegas. Those days are gone for good. Who wants to imagine Elvis at eighty? Elvis at forty-two was cringe-worthy enough.

But for many years after 1977, when his death was reported, there were silly conspiracy theories that he was still alive. In the early 1990s I got solid confirmation that Elvis was indeed dead.

I was asked to give Grand Rounds, a formal medical lecture, at Baptist Memorial Hospital in Memphis, Tennessee. Old Baptist is long gone now, demolished years ago, but it was one of those landmark American hospitals like Cook County with a venerable medical tradition. Built in the early part of the twentieth century, it was a hospital for indigent patients and one of the most important training hospitals for nurses and doctors in the United States for over half a century.

The most famous patient that Baptist ever cared for came in or, more accurately, was wheeled in, on August 16, 1977. That afternoon Elvis Presley, the King, was transported in full cardiac arrest from his Graceland mansion to the Baptist emergency room.

To this day, the cause of his cardiac arrest remains a subject of contention. Was it due to the combination of painkillers, soporifics, tranquilizers, and mood stabilizers in his system, or the ill effects on his heart of homemade biscuits fried in butter, sausage patties, scrambled eggs, and lots of bacon? Most likely the drugs and diet were both to blame.

Whatever the cause, after long and harrowing resuscitation attempts by the Baptist staff, Elvis was pronounced dead. Ever since that day, for a week in mid-August, people still come from all over the world to visit his final resting place at the family mansion at Graceland, sort of a rock 'n' roll pilgrimage. Some of these sojourners are the grandchildren of the teenage rebels who listened to him or watched him on *The Ed Sullivan Show* in the 1950s.

For many years after his death there were Elvis sightings. It was said he'd given up performing, faked his death, and moved to Hawaii. Or he was spotted munching a Whopper with cheese at a Burger King outside of Kalamazoo, Michigan. Hawaii is understandable, but why he would be outside Kalamazoo was anyone's guess. However, the "munching a Whopper" part of the story does lend a certain air of credibility to that particular account.

When you give Grand Rounds as a visiting doctor, one of the rituals you must go through is dining with important members of the medical staff before the lecture. My Grand Rounds was no exception, and I had an early morning breakfast with some of the medical honchos, including the doctor in charge of coordinating the event.

He was an amiable Southern gentleman with a beautiful Mississippi drawl, the kind with which every sentence ends with an inflection that sounds like a question. As a true man of the South, he referred to me as a "Yankee," but without any trace of enmity over the long-ago war. What's done is done.

The hospitality was unmistakable. We dined on grits—not my standard breakfast fare, but it was the South, after all, and it would be rude to refuse.

Initially, the conversation was strictly medical—the latest treatment for this or that, or the current thinking about some journal article. Except for my host's beautiful Southern lilt, the conversation seemed rather mundane until he dropped a small tidbit unobtrusively into the conversation. I forget how it came up, but he told me—quite matter-of-factly, no bragging—that fifteen years before he had been the senior doctor in the emergency room the day they brought Elvis in. He was in charge of resuscitating him, and when the resuscitation failed, it was his job to pronounce Elvis dead.

It had never occurred to me that someone actually did that. Logically, of course, someone had to. I had been in charge of hundreds of resuscitations and pronounced many people dead, but never a celebrity, and certainly never anyone as big as the King.

At that moment this Southern doctor became a special person in my eyes. I dropped my jaw and my grits spoon as well. As an Elvis fan, I have been to Graceland three times (I highly recommend a visit, especially to the Jungle Room), though never during Elvis Week. Now here I was with the man who could answer the question, once and for all, of whether Elvis was really dead.

I stammered, "I have to know two things. Was it really Elvis and was he really dead?"

Clearly this was not the first time he had been asked. I think he had an answer prepared for this inquisitive Yankee. He stopped eating his grits and looked me in the eye. His visage turned serious and with that Southern drawl he answered, "I'm not gon' lie to ya. It was sho'nuff Elvis."

Then he paused a second for emphasis.

"An' they don't come any deaduh."

For me, that settled it once and for all. Elvis was dead.

But the doctor wasn't finished. He resumed eating and then told me how the very next day, some tabloid had offered $25,000 to anyone—doctors, nurses, X-ray technicians—who was in the emergency room when Elvis was brought in, to tell their story. The hospital administration had gotten wind of the offer. The doctor looked me in the eye again, but now his expression was more one of amusement.

"The hospital put out a memo for the whole staff. And it said y'all can talk to the newspaper people. Be our guest. Jes' consider that $25,000 your sev'rance pay from Baptist." No one talked to the reporters.

I thought about asking him if he knew what Elvis died of, whether it was the drugs or a heart attack, but I could tell he considered the subject closed right then and there. As if all those years later perhaps that severance threat was still hanging over his head.

15

THE DUKE OF SPAIN AND THE PROFESSOR FROM PENN

"For my part, answer'd Don Quixote, I will hear you attentively."

—MIGUEL DE CERVANTES, *DON QUIXOTE*

THERE IS A famous story, perhaps apocryphal, of an elderly, experienced pediatrician who practiced in the days when doctors made house calls. He was summoned to the home of a family with six children, and all were manifesting the same symptoms. After attending a church picnic the previous day, they all had fevers and suffered from abdominal pain. The doctor examined each child and informed the parents, "These five children have food poisoning. The sixth one has appendicitis." His diagnosis of appendicitis was borne out when the sixth child was taken to the hospital and had surgery.

The point of the story is that in medicine, what appears to be self-evident may not be true. The initial evaluation of a patient means assessing how she looks, how she talks, and the nature of her demeanor. The first impression created by this information can be mistaken, to the detriment of the patient. The inexperienced and the careless often rely too heavily on first impressions without attempting to obtain a fuller picture; this was the lesson provided by the elderly pediatrician.

My father taught me that same lesson by recounting the long-ago story of a disheveled, inebriated man brought into County with a cut on his head. He was seen in the emergency room, his head wound was deemed superficial, and the doctors sutured it up and then admitted him. In the '50s, it was not unusual for inebriated patients to be admitted to the hospital to sober up and to be observed for other complications of alcoholism. Today, in the brave new world of medicine, hospital administrators, insurance companies, and the government all frown on such "frivolous" medical admissions.

The drunken man was sent to a large open ward, with many similar patients. The majority of them were denizens of Chicago's Skid Row, an area of Madison Street where thousands of down-on-their-luck alcoholics lived in flophouses, drank cheap liquor, and transmitted tuberculosis and other communicable diseases to one another. (The term "skid row" isn't heard much anymore; in many cities these areas have been cleaned up and gentrified. In New York, the equivalent neighborhood was the Bowery in Lower Manhattan.) When those down-and-outers got too drunk, started coughing up blood, or got mixed up in scrapes, the police or the ambulances would bring them to County, which was only about a mile away. Many of them knew each other, and when they were on a large open ward together, it was something of a Skid Row revival meeting.

There was little to suggest this particular rumpled little man was anything but another one of these unfortunates. The police wagon that brought him in came from the Madison Street district, where the man was found wandering aimlessly. He slept off his alcoholic stupor, and in the morning he washed up and shaved in the common bathroom of the hospital ward. But there were two things about him that were at least slightly unusual. The first was that he barely spoke any English.

The second was something the doctors and nurses failed to notice: the clothes he wore when he was brought to the hospital. After he was admitted, he was issued the standard hospital gown. However, in the plastic bag that accompanied him upstairs was a much nicer outfit than that of the typical Madison Street crowd. No one opened the plastic bag containing his clothes, but if they did, they would have noticed that his slacks, though bloodstained from his wound, were neatly tapered. His collared shirt was not the typical three-dollar throwaway that so many of the alcoholics wore (if they wore a collared shirt at all; many wore T-shirts instead). His shoes were expensive. And he had a scarf; scarves were hardly de rigueur on Madison Street. But his clothes, in the portable dresser next to his bed, remained unexamined.

When the doctors made rounds the next morning, they walked to each bed and checked the patients, most of whom were in various states of alcohol withdrawal. Some were just hungover; a couple were in worse shape. When the doctors came to that man's bed, he was chattering away furiously in Spanish, punctuated by an occasional English phrase. He kept exclaiming he was the Duke of Spain. In those days, there were no Spanish translators to verify his claim.

Alcoholics in withdrawal commonly fabricate some grandiose new identity, so his statement, "I AM THE DUKE OF SPAIN!" seemed to just confirm that this was someone in the throes of withdrawal. Yet as the day went on, the man pleaded to the nurses even more vociferously that he was the Duke of Spain. They paid him no mind.

"I AM THE DUKE OF SPAIN!"

This continued for three days before the doctors started wondering what exactly was going on with the chattering man. Though most likely delusional, he demonstrated no other symptoms of alcoholism. The other problem was that his bloodwork failed to support the diagnosis of chronic alcoholism. He was becoming a medical mystery.

"I AM THE DUKE OF SPAIN!"

The next day, the mystery was cleared up when some Chicago police officers came to the ward, accompanied by officials from the Spanish consulate. For days, the police had been looking for him; now they had found him at County Hospital.

The chattering man really was the Duke of Spain, or at least *a* duke of some province in Spain. He was apparently part of a group of Spanish noblemen who had stopped in Chicago while on a cross-country train trip.

In the early 1950s, before jet travel was common, most people traveling from New York to Los Angeles went by train. This included Europeans with business on the West Coast, who would cross the Atlantic on RMS *Queen Mary*, the SS *United States*, or the French Line's SS *Liberté*. In New York, they would book on through a Pullman car to Los Angeles (think Cary Grant and Eva Marie Saint in Hitchcock's *North by Northwest*). This meant overnighting to Chicago on the 20th Century Ltd. or the Broadway Ltd., and there would always be time to kill in downtown Chicago during the day before the Super Chief left for the West Coast in the evening.

The duke and his companions had arrived aboard the 20th Century Ltd. Maybe he had a few too many cocktails on the train. Whatever happened, he probably stopped to have a few more drinks somewhere around the LaSalle Street Station, perhaps one of the downtown hotel bars. He wandered away from the train near Madison Street, only a couple of blocks away. He fell and hit his head (or perhaps someone hit him), and when the police found him, he was inebriated and bleeding in the street. *Time to take another Madison Street drunk to County.*

At the hospital, the doctors had the same initial impression and made the same misidentification. And because he couldn't speak much English, he couldn't tell them anything other than "I AM THE DUKE OF SPAIN!"

And, sure enough, he was.

A similar thing happened when I was the senior attending on the tuberculosis service at County. During our rounds, we came to the isolation rooms where patients with active tuberculosis were treated while they were still considered contagious.

These isolation rooms were depressing and dark, and the patients were alone most of the time. Visitors, nurses, and doctors had to don masks and gowns before entering, which only reinforced the patients' feeling of isolation. In most cases, these patients had few relatives and no one who cared to spend much time with them. The patients couldn't leave their rooms and there were no televisions to watch. Some had portable radios, which represented their only contact with the outside world.

Many of these patients were malnourished alcoholics from Skid Row, who drank alone in their rooms or with other residents of the same cheap hotel. The heavy alcohol consumption weakened their immune systems and they infected each other with tuberculosis. Eventually, they became so weak that they could barely walk, and this would bring them to the hospital for treatment. Most of them were gentle people who had always existed on the fringes of society. They escaped from the world through alcohol. For the most part, they were pitiable characters.

Mr. Jones was one of those, or so I thought.

He was a small white man in his late forties with long, stringy gray hair that made him look twenty years older. No teeth and a deathly pallor. When you walked into the dark room that was barely illuminated by the light from his window, you noticed how thin he was (the medical term is *cachexia*). Between malnourishment and tuberculosis, he weighed less than a hundred pounds. He coughed continually into a paper cup next to his bed. It looked as though he hadn't been on his feet for days. The scene was reminiscent of a Hieronymus Bosch painting.

When we came into his room, he met us with a pair of eyes as sad and forlorn as any I'd ever seen. He didn't appear to have much time left.

I was not paying close attention to the residents as they questioned him. They treated him as simply one more poor Skid Row alcoholic with tuberculosis. And, in truth, there was very little reason to believe otherwise. But everyone has story, and in medicine things are not always what they seem.

As the residents and I were leaving the room, I happened to notice a book by his bedside, *The Decline and Fall of the Roman Empire* by Edward Gibbon. Not exactly the book you would expect to see on the night table of an alcoholic from Skid Row. I sent the residents ahead and went back to talk to Mr. Jones.

"Mr. Jones, I just wanted to ask you something."

"Sure, Doc. What is it?"

"That book by your bedside. Are you reading it?"

"Oh, I've read it before. But it's my favorite, so I like to look at it when I have time. And you may have noticed I have a lot of time."

He didn't sound like the typical County tuberculosis patient.

"Mr. Jones, how did you get here?"

Then he told an amazing story.

"I was a history professor at the University of Pennsylvania for fifteen years."

That made him the most educated person in the room when we visited him on rounds, me included. He continued, "I drank at Penn, but I wouldn't say I had a drinking problem. It never interfered with my teaching."

"What happened?"

"My daughter died of leukemia. Six months later, my wife and son were killed when a drunk driver hit them from behind and they smashed into a train. So I lost everything I had in six months. I just figured what was the point, you know? I quit my teaching job at Penn, left Philadelphia, came to Chicago, and started drinking heavily. Ten years now. I've been arrested a couple of times, blew through most of my money, and wound up on Madison Street. If it wasn't for tuberculosis, I'd still be over there in my room drinking. No one bothers you there."

"Don't you have any other relatives?"

He laughed. His expression suggested there was another story there, perhaps family issues, but it really wasn't my place to probe. Before I left, I asked just one more question.

"Is *The Decline and Fall of the Roman Empire* a good book?"

He smiled enigmatically.

"None better. You should try it sometime. I'd give you my copy but, well, there really isn't much else to do here. You know they don't let you drink in your room." It was his attempt at levity.

Then he broke into a coughing fit, waved to me, and I left his room. That was a Friday, and I had the weekend off. When I returned on Monday, his room was empty. I knew what had happened to him, but I asked what became of the copy of Gibbon on his nightstand. No one knew. Like him, it was gone forever.

16

WEST SIDE DRAMA
IN THREE PARTS

"Fate and history never seem to work in orderly ways.
Timings are unpredictable and do not wait
upon conveniences."

—MICHAEL ARIS

FOR DECADES, THE four hospitals and their ancillary clinics located within a mile of each other on the West Side of Chicago cared for more patients than any other medical complex in North America. The West Side Medical Center, as it was known, is no longer the country's largest, but thousands of people still pass in and out of the neighborhood every day. Interesting interactions among so many people, rich and poor, sick and healthy, happen not only in the hospitals but outside as well. No matter where you walk, there is a story. One day, for me, the story was a traditional drama in three parts, complete with setup, confrontation, and resolution.

Act I (Setup): One afternoon, an elderly man was walking back and forth just outside County Hospital. He appeared to be looking for something or someone. I noticed him pacing as I left the hospital.

His unusual behavior singled him out and I paused to observe him for a few minutes. Most people who leave the hospital face forward, because they are waiting for a bus, a taxi, or someone to take them home. But this man kept looking back at the hospital. He seemed to be studying the building itself.

People kept bumping into or brushing by him, but he seemed not to notice. He appeared to be completely oblivious to the minor irritation he was creating. Every few seconds he would move to another angle for a different view of the hospital. He seemed quite confused by what he was looking at. He wasn't the only one confused; after watching him for several minutes, I was completely bewildered. I couldn't figure out what he was doing.

Finally I approached him.

"Excuse me, sir. You look lost. Can I help you get somewhere?"

He gave me a gruff look and confronted me with a staccato patter, "I'm looking for the address of this place. Where is it? Why isn't it on the front of the goddam building? Do you know the address of this place?"

I was taken aback and answered, "This is the county hospital. You know, Cook County Hospital."

This did nothing to mollify him. If anything, it enraged him.

"I *KNOW* it's the fucking Cook County Hospital. *WHAT'S THE ADDRESS?*"

He began shouting, and a crowd was forming. His demeanor made it appear as though our confrontation was a hostile one. It must have looked like I was harassing the old man. That's not a good thing, so I tried to de-escalate the situation. I still didn't have a good idea of what was going on, but I was trying to appear helpful. Actually, even though I'd worked at the hospital for years, I wasn't sure of the address myself.

"Let me go in and ask the woman at information."

After getting the address at the front desk, I came outside and told him, "The hospital address is 1835 West Harrison." I also gave him a card with the address on it. This seemed to placate him.

He repeated the address, "1835 West Harrison Street. That's good to know."

The crowd, hoping for a show and not getting one, dispersed. Still, I was curious as he kept repeating the address to himself, sotto voce.

"I'm just curious, sir. Why is it so important to you to know the address?"

He glared at me. "Listen, you know what they do every time I come in this goddamn place? The first thing they ask me is 'Do you know where you are?' Well, from now on, I'm going to tell them: 1835 West Harrison."

Only on the West Side of Chicago.

Act II (Confrontation): After I left the hospital on foot, I had to wait at a long stoplight on a busy street to make it to my car. While I was waiting, a large black man with an angry expression came up next to me. He may have been six foot six, 250 pounds, and he seemed to eye me suspiciously as we both waited for the light to change. Perhaps it was just in my mind, but there was a hint of menace about him as he scowled at me. I had maybe another thirty seconds of discomfort before the light would change and allow me to remove myself from the situation. For me, at least, it was somewhat tense.

It was right after Halloween, and I happened to have a couple of bite-size candy bars in my pocket. I fingered my pocket nervously and I came up with some mini Snickers bars. Seeking to defuse the tension at the long stoplight, I pulled them out of my pocket, made eye contact with him, smiled, and offered him the candy bars. I didn't know how he would react to my peace offering.

For a brief moment, he looked at me quizzically. He accepted the candy and the scowl left his face. He didn't say anything, but I thought the tension was broken.

It was, but I was mistaken in believing the encounter was over.

Before the light changed, he immediately dug into his pocket and came up with a bunch of bite size Milky Way bars. What were the chances of that? Without a word, he offered them to me. Surprised, I took them graciously. In unspoken terms, he was responding to my peace offering, and his was an offering of friendship.

After taking his mini Milky Way bars, I nodded to him in thanks, and a barely perceptible smile appeared on his face. There was an element of humor in the episode. We crossed the street together and then went our separate ways. Not a word was ever spoken between us.

To an outsider, the whole exchange, which lasted no more than half a minute, might have appeared to be scripted. To a visitor from another planet, this mini chocolate swap might have looked like a greeting ritual from some unfamiliar culture. But there on Ashland Avenue, one of the busiest streets in Chicago, it was just a brief, mutual expression of humanity and friendship, courtesy of the Mars candy company.

Only on the West Side of Chicago.

Act III (Resolution): That should have been the end of the day's drama, but part three happened that night, when I picked up three of my friends with tickets to go to a Chicago Bulls game at the old Chicago Stadium. Back in the early 1990s, before the stadium was torn down to build the new United Center, the Bulls had Michael Jordan and were the hottest ticket in town, having won a couple of championships.

The old stadium had plenty of charm and character, but one of the things it did not have was convenient parking. When the Bulls were popular, there was usually a traffic jam around the facility; cars would wait for half an hour just to get into a parking lot. Failure to account for this when leaving for the game would probably mean a late arrival.

The stadium was only a mile away from the hospital (1835 West Harrison, in case you have forgotten) but it was in a bad neighborhood. Today, much of that neighborhood has been revitalized, and the popularity of the Bulls and Blackhawks has made the area much safer. But in those days it was unwise to stray more than a block or two from the stadium. There was a lot of crime. Many young doctors in the medical center received their trauma experience working on patients brought from that nearby neighborhood.

On this night, I was the driver, and I was late picking everyone up. Sure enough, we got caught in the parking traffic. Actually, we were not sitting in traffic—we *were* the traffic. The game was due to start in ten minutes. We were no more than a block and a half from the stadium, but with the traffic jam, it looked like we might miss the first quarter, if not the first half. Bulls tickets were hard to come by, and I was blowing it. My friends were not pleased with the fact that I was late and there was nothing I could do but sit in that traffic helplessly, watching cars creep into the lot in single file.

The atmosphere in the car was frosty when one of my passengers—at this point I wasn't sure they were still my friends—said acerbically, "You realize you will be paying when we get into the lot."

This was clearly a breach of our usual etiquette; parking fees were typically covered, at least in part, by the passengers. But with the game five minutes away, I was in no position to quarrel. So on top of everything else, I would be out the twenty dollars for parking. It appeared that the highlight of my day was the candy exchange outside County.

Suddenly, a young black man approached my driver's side window and tapped. He seemed to be trying to get us to park in his yard, off the street right where we were stuck. It was worth a try even if it might cost five or ten dollars more—I didn't plan to haggle over price. There was, of course, the question of how secure the car would be in his yard (and how secure we would be retrieving it afterwards). The lighting was dim and the yard looked ominous. I was weighing these factors in my mind as I assessed the situation.

The clock was ticking, Jordan was warming up, the game would be starting any minute and I had three former friends staring daggers at me.

I was desperate.

I rolled down my window.

"How much?"

He gave me a look and grinned.

"Dr. Franklin? For you? Are you kidding? You just come right in here. We'll put you where you can get out right away after the game."

What was he talking about? I was confused but he cleared up the confusion immediately when he called out to his friends in the yard.

"Yo, guys. This is Dr. Franklin. He's my mom's doctor. He's a good guy. Give him our number-one spot." He turned back to me and said, "No charge for you."

My passengers were stunned at this dramatic reversal of fortune. One minute before we'd been in a long line, and now we had a great parking spot for free. As a gesture of thanks, I gave each of the guys in the yard a five-dollar bill. A rescue never came cheaper.

"Dr. Franklin, the mayor's car won't get better attention. Even Michael's car won't get better attention. Now you guys get in there. Game is starting in five minutes."

For that crucial five minutes, I was the most important guy on the West Side of Chicago, at least other than Michael Jordan.

We made it in time for tip-off. And my friends—they were my friends again—were never as impressed with me as they were that evening.

Only on the West Side of Chicago.

17

MR. RODRIGUEZ'S SECRET, AND THE ASSASSIN'S VICTIM

_____

"The proper study of Mankind is Man."

—ALEXANDER POPE

ONE OF THE greatest joys of working in medicine is meeting unforgettable patients. Some of their names and their stories still resonate decades later. As an internist, I actually felt sorry for some of my professional colleagues who went into fields such as radiology, anesthesia, and pathology. They may have had fantastically stimulating and lucrative careers, and they certainly helped save lives and relieve suffering with their skills, but the nature of their work never allowed them to bond with patients and hear their stories.

For a few years in the early 1980s, I had to do rounds at a Veterans Administration hospital. VA hospitals are a crucial part of the US military system, charged with caring for American veterans of all our past wars. Recently, the hospitals have been maligned—sometimes fairly, sometimes not—for the quality of the care they deliver. The system has upgraded its record-keeping and care procedures since I worked there, but back then there always seemed to be some veterans slipping through the cracks. Well, I never saw anyone slip through the cracks like Mr. Rodriguez.

One day I was making rounds with my residents and students on the medical ward at the VA. We came to the room of a very old man, Mr. Rodriguez. No one knew exactly when he was born; his chart said the date of his birth was "1/1/00," or January 1, 1900. That would have put him in his early eighties, but he certainly appeared older than that. The resident presenting Mr. Rodriguez's case at bedside claimed he was eighty-two. When I asked the resident how he knew that, he told me he was going by the computer default date of the patient's birth. If it comes from the computer and is on the chart, it must be right.

Considering how old Mr. Rodriguez looked, he was somewhat frail but reasonably healthy. He spoke English hesitatingly. After the resident finished his presentation, I put the question directly to Mr. Rodriguez of how old he was. He was vague and told me he was born sometime in the 1880s, so he was actually closer to one hundred. Back then, we didn't see many patients who were that old; centenarians are far more common today than they were then. After a few more innocuous questions from the residents I examined him and talked with him about his health problems, which were not serious, and then we were about to leave.

But there was something intriguing about him. Every patient has a backstory, and those at the VA are often the most compelling, though they are often left untold. Some of these men were war heroes; many had shown uncommon bravery in their youth. Most of the residents, and many of the attendings, are under thirty-five and have never spent any time in the military. There is a pernicious tendency on the part of some of the younger doctors to patronize the older veterans. Perhaps nowhere in our health care system is there is a greater disconnect between patient and caregiver than at the VA, and that may account for some of the problems with its system.

In the days before the Iraq and Afghanistan conflicts, most of our patients were veterans of either World War II or Korea, with a smaller number from Vietnam. Occasionally we would care for a World War I vet, but most of them had died by the early 1980s (the last American World War I vet, Frank Buckles, died in 2011 at the age of 110). Mr. Rodriguez, if he was born in the 1880s, was definitely too old to have been a World War II vet. A quick bit of mental math suggested he would have been in his thirties when America entered World War I. A little old for a doughboy, but maybe he enlisted late. I felt compelled to ask him.

"Mr. Rodriguez, you couldn't have been in World War II. Were you in World War I?"

"No."

I was puzzled. "Where did you serve?"

"The Spanish-American War."

That was a bit of a shock; he fought in a war that began in the nineteenth century. For all of us, that was a distant page out of the history books. *Remember the Maine.*

He was certainly the first Spanish-American War veteran anyone in the room—including me—had ever seen. I have to admit I was impressed. I turned to the assembled medical personnel and said, "Ladies and gentlemen, Mr. Rodriguez is part of history. He is probably the only Spanish-American War vet you will ever take care of."

Mr. Rodriguez seemed nonplussed by the distinction I conferred upon him. It bothered him that we were speaking about it. Then he motioned me over to lean close to him so he could whisper in my ear. Whatever he was about to tell me, he didn't want the rest of the group to hear.

He repeated, "Spanish-American War."

Then, in a barely audible voice, he said, "Spanish side."

Mr. Rodriguez was indeed a veteran of the Spanish-American War; it's just that he had fought for Spain.

He put his finger up to his mouth indicating it was a secret and should remain a secret. Neither he nor I had any idea what would happen if the people at the hospital found out. Perhaps they would kick him out of the hospital. It wasn't in the VA mission to take care of enemy veterans, even nineteenth-century enemy veterans. I winked and put my finger to my lips as a signal that his secret was safe with me. Time to go.

"All right, team, let's finish up rounds."

I waved to Mr. Rodriguez. "Take care, Mr. Rodriguez."

When rounds were over, I sent the residents and students on their way to do their work. Meanwhile, I hung around the nurses' station for a few minutes, chuckling to myself about my Spanish-American War vet.

Just then, a young social worker came by. I wondered if she knew Mr. Rodriguez's secret. I called her over. The social workers had access to the patients' service records and usually knew their histories.

I asked, "You know Mr. Rodriguez, the guy in 314?"

"Oh yes. Isn't he a sweet old man?"

I was getting the impression she didn't know, but I decided to push the issue a little.

"He seems like a nice old guy. But I was wondering about his service history. What's the deal? When did he fight?"

She laughed, "Well, you know he fought in the Spanish-American War. And it's a funny thing but we can't find his service records. We figure the records for those vets could be anywhere, so we just let it go. We don't have any other Spanish-American vets so he's sort of a celebrity. We're not making a big deal about his service history."

It sounded like a line out of *Catch-22*, but I could tell from her earnest look she didn't know he was an enemy veteran.

"That's nice," I said. "Uncle Sugar."

"Uncle Sugar" was a semisarcastic variant of "Uncle Sam." It was the term we used when the government did something nice for a veteran. I never saw Mr. Rodriguez again, but I did not let on. His secret was safe with me.

———————

Another one of my most memorable patients was Darryl Stingley, a well-known athlete from Chicago, whom I met when I was on a rotation at the Rehabilitation Institute. He was a professional football player, but I had heard of him long before that because he'd been something of a high school legend. Spectators and television viewers may be aware of the violence in football, but not the true elemental level of the game's danger. As a physician and fan, I learned this firsthand from Darryl Stingley.

In the 1960s, Stingley was a talented running back from Marshall High School, in one of Chicago's most dangerous neighborhoods. I followed his career safely from the distance of the bucolic suburbs. Lithe and fast, Stingley escaped the mean streets of the West Side when he was recruited to play football at Purdue. The coaches, impressed with his speed, converted Stingley from running back to wide receiver, since they had another powerful running back, Otis Armstrong, who was also from inner city Chicago. Both men went on to have wonderful careers, first at Purdue and then in the NFL. Stingley was a New England Patriots first-round draft choice and became a top NFL receiver, while Armstrong became a star for the Denver Broncos.

One particular college game bears mention. In Stingley's senior year at Purdue, I was one of 105,000 people watching at Michigan Stadium when Purdue played Michigan, then ranked number three in the country. An upset would put Purdue in line for a Rose Bowl berth, something unheard of in the early 1970s, when the Rose Bowl was the exclusive domain of Michigan and Ohio State. Stingley and Armstrong were only two of Purdue's stars; the Boilermakers also had quarterback Gary Danielson, the future TV announcer, and Dave Butz, who became a Hall of Fame lineman for the Washington Redskins.

Purdue actually outplayed Michigan but lost when Armstrong, who had a clear path to the end zone for the potential game-winning touchdown, slipped on the artificial turf deep in Michigan territory. That key play occurred right in front of where I was sitting. The Boilermakers lost by three points, dashing their Rose Bowl hopes. It was a crushing defeat for a talented team.

Five years after that, when he was in the NFL, Darryl Stingley's life changed forever owing to a tackle by Jack Tatum, an Oakland Raiders defensive back. The backstory on Tatum was that in high school he was named one of New Jersey's top ten defensive players of the century. He went on to Ohio State, and the Buckeyes won a National Championship with Tatum anchoring the defense. Tatum was a two-year All-American and 1970 College Defensive Player of the Year, with a reputation as a vicious hitter who inspired fear in wide receivers. Not surprisingly, he became part of Al Davis's 1970s Oakland Raiders. Davis, a tough Brooklyn kid, molded the Raiders in his image, fierce and intimidating. Tatum's fearsome hits, and his nom de guerre, "the Assassin," burnished that image. Tatum's Raiders won two Super Bowls and might have won a third but for the irony that Tatum's crushing hit on a Pittsburgh receiver allowed Steeler Franco Harris to make the famous Immaculate Reception that beat Oakland in a last-minute miracle.

The game in which Stingley and Tatum crossed paths, literally, was a meaningless 1978 exhibition game. Stingley went for a pass over the middle and Tatum unleashed a savage hit on the defenseless receiver, fracturing two of Stingley's cervical vertebrae and leaving him quadriplegic. No penalty was called. Patriots coach Chuck Fairbanks said, "I saw replays many times, and many times Jack Tatum was criticized. But there wasn't anything at that time illegal about that play." Today, Tatum would probably be fined and suspended.

"It was one of those things that happens everyone regrets," Gene Upshaw, Tatum's teammate, said. "I know a lot of people in New England think differently, but Jack had no intention of hurting him. I saw him hit people like that lots of times. That was the way he played." Stingley's injury motivated Upshaw, then director of the NFL Players Association, to provide benefits to disabled players.

Stingley was wheelchair bound after the hit, and he spent some time at the Rehabilitation Institute of Chicago, where I took care of him as a senior medical student. The muscular athlete I remembered was now small, his physique atrophied and contorted in his motorized chair. Some of the kids he grew up with were patients there also, victims of spinal trauma from the neighborhood gunfire that he had managed to escape.

One day I mentioned to him that I followed his career from Marshall to Purdue. I told him I was at the Michigan game in which the Rose Bowl hung in the balance. He remembered the game of course, and smiled perceptibly with a nod that said, "We should have won that one."

John Madden, the famous announcer who was the Raiders' coach that fateful day when Stingley was injured, made Darryl Stingley an honorary Raider, always to be treated as such. It was a gracious gesture as a follow-up to one of the most horrific injuries in NFL history. During Madden's Pro Football Hall of Fame induction speech, he even referred to Stingley: "We all like to see a hard, aggressive play, but you always want the guy to get up."

Jack Tatum played several more years after the Stingley hit, but he was never the same player after that. The Stingley play took some of his aggressiveness away. By most accounts, he was a decent person off the field, but he will always carry the legacy of the villain in the Stingley story. He didn't help his cause when he wrote books after his career was over, relishing his reputation as a football assassin and never showing contrition.

Both those superb athletes died young. Jack Tatum died at sixty-one from complications of diabetes and Darryl Stingley died at fifty-five from complications of paralysis.

When he learned that Jack Tatum, who never apologized to him, had his own leg amputated because of diabetes later in life, Stingley said, "You can't, as a human being, feel happy about something like that happening to another human being. Maybe the natural reaction is to think he got what was coming to him, but I don't accept human nature as our real nature. Human nature teaches us to hate. God teaches us to love."

I saw Darryl Stingley once more, this time at a Chicago Bulls game. Courtside in his wheelchair, he made eye contact with me in the stands. He evidently remembered me caring for him many years earlier and I think he mouthed "Michigan game." There was amazing spirit and resolve in him. He married, had children, and started a charitable foundation in Chicago. I met few patients in my career who showed as much character as Darryl Stingley.

18

OF PRESIDENTS, NEGRO LEAGUERS, SERIAL KILLERS, AND LINDA DARNELL

"Oh, celluloid heroes never feel any pain.
Oh, celluloid heroes never really die."

—THE KINKS

E VERY DOCTOR I'VE ever met likes to name-drop about caring for famous people at one time or another. Whether they admit it or not, most doctors enjoy bragging about their celebrity patients. Often, especially when the patient is a politician, the doctor is limited by confidentiality, but if it's a prominent athlete or a movie star, doctors like to tell their friends in private, even if the relationship cannot be made public. Of course, the chances of having a famous patient are far greater in some places than others. Plastic surgeons in West L.A. and cardiologists in Manhattan are much more likely to have prominent patients than are practitioners in rural Montana.

If the celebrity gives consent, the doctor may even use him or her as advertising. In recent years, there has sometimes been a trend for doctors, especially orthopedic surgeons and internists, to pay large sums to be affiliated with a professional sports team. It's often a wise business decision; the doctors can more than make back the money they pay the team, since patients with knee injuries or hip problems naturally want to be treated by their local team's famous orthopedist.

Of course, if something goes wrong with the celebrity's treatment, this can backfire. This happened on national television to the Washington Redskins' orthopedic surgeon, Dr. James Andrews. Regarded by many as the top orthopedic surgeon in North America, he suffered a blow to his reputation when he failed to intervene in a playoff game to keep a visibly injured Robert Griffin III, Washington's star quarterback, from reentering the game. Several plays later, Griffin suffered a career-threatening injury. It's hard being a doctor before eighty thousand people and a national television audience, even for the best of orthopedic surgeons.

The biggest celebrity I *almost* treated was President Reagan. I had worked at the George Washington Medical Center in DC the year before the president was elected, and I'd had to make a choice between doing postgraduate intensive care training there or at University Hospital in Cleveland. At the last moment I had chosen Cleveland. Had I done my training at George Washington, I thought, I would have been working in the intensive care unit when President Reagan was taken there after he was shot in 1981. As I watched the television coverage of the assassination attempt, I mused about what might have been.

Soon afterward I was disabused of this notion. I saw some people from George Washington and mentioned that I might have been on the team taking care of the president if I had decided to work there.

One of them said to me, "Are you kidding? You would have been the junior person on the team. You wouldn't have come within a mile of the president. You would have needed a telescope to get a look at him."

Well, then maybe I would have taken care of wounded press secretary James Brady.

When you work at a prestigious medical center, you might get a chance to take care of a celebrity, but at County Hospital there just aren't that many famous people who come in. But some infamous ones have been brought there involuntarily, and there is an ethical issue involved with caring for the notorious patient. This dilemma was illustrated graphically in 2013 at Boston's Beth Israel Deaconess Medical Center. When the accused Boston Marathon bomber Dzhokhar Tsarnaev was brought bleeding and wounded into the emergency room, the staff faced a distressing predicament. How would the nurses and physicians feel about taking care of such a patient, one whose values are inimical to society? As one trauma nurse who cared for Tsarnaev during his first night in the hospital explained to the *Boston Globe*, "I am compassionate, that's what we do. But should I be? The rest of the world hates him right now. The emotions are like one big salad, all tossed around." Everyone who treated Tsarnaev will struggle with such emotions for a long time.

Health care professionals in emergency rooms and intensive care units must sometimes treat felons, murderers, and rapists. They don't have the luxury of refusing to treat a patient, no matter how odious that person may be. When something like the Boston bombing happens, the usual approach is to view the offender as simply another patient, just part of the hospital routine. While that may be an adequate defense mechanism in treating most criminals, it becomes more complicated in treating particularly heinous suspects—in this case an alleged terrorist. Many in the public ask caregivers, "How can you take care of that person? Why do you do it?"

The short, but incomplete, answer is part of the code nurses and physicians live by. But in reality, caring for patients like Tsarnaev compels even the most hardened nurse or physician to undergo some uncomfortable introspection. As that Boston trauma nurse added, "You see a hurt nineteen-year-old and you can't help but feel sorry for him." Yet she said

she "would not be upset if he got the death penalty. There is no way to rec-
oncile the two different feelings." I have heard similar sentiments expressed
by military physicians who cared for enemy prisoners of war.

That internal conflict can be difficult to manage when you work in a
hospital, especially when you are tasked with saving the life or relieving
the pain of someone who has maliciously taken innocent lives or caused
others to suffer undeservedly. Moreover, the constraints of confidentiality
often prohibit caregivers from discussing outside the hospital the care they
give to a high-profile patient. Not being able to share your feelings about
treating the subject of headlines across the whole country, or the whole
world, can be stressful.

One final thing about caring for notorious patients like Tsarnaev: there
is something about them that will always be etched in your memory. Doctors and nurses generally forget the vast majority of the patients they treat
in the course of their professional careers. But not in cases like this. No
doctor or nurse at Beth Israel is likely to forget Tsarnaev. Each may have
a different memory of some specific detail about treating him, but those
details will remain with the caregivers for the rest of their lives.

A physician I knew once cared for a notorious convicted murderer who
tortured his victims before killing them. Years later, my colleague was able
to describe, in vivid detail, the fear this murderer had of needles—the irony
of a sadistic killer who could not bear the smallest needle for a tetanus shot
or to have his blood drawn.

For me, it was the faces. Many years ago, I briefly treated several people
convicted of particularly gruesome crimes. All have been dead for many
years, but each made national headlines in their day. Even today, decades
later, I remember how each would stare at me menacingly when I came
near them.

I was the first doctor to see serial killer John Wayne Gacy when he was
apprehended. Minutes after his arrest he was brought to a highly guarded
isolation cell at the Cook County Jail, where I was working the medical
detail. All I had to do was renew a prescription for a medicine he was tak-

ing. But I did have to come to his cell in the middle of the night. As he sat there mute, he stared right at me. In recalling the episode, I am reminded of Hannibal Lecter in *Silence of the Lambs*—in other words, it was one of those situations you want to extricate yourself from as quickly as possible. That stare will never leave me.

I also treated notorious mass murderer Richard Speck shortly before his death. Speck had killed eight student nurses on the South Side of Chicago in 1966. There was an odd convergence between my story and Speck's. As a twelve-year-old newspaper delivery boy, my first day on the job was the day the story of the Speck murders broke. So I began my new occupation by delivering newspapers with headlines of Speck's crime to people's lawns (and occasionally to their roofs).

Twenty-five years later, the man who was responsible for those head-lines was my patient at County. By the time I treated Speck, a contempt-ible character to begin with, he was a different person from the murderer of 1966. His rough face was transformed by the female hormones he had taken in prison. He looked completely different, with hormone-enhanced breasts and female features. It's another thing I will never forget.

The convergence was not simply between Speck and me but also between Speck and County Hospital. After Speck murdered the nurses, there was a nationwide manhunt for the then-unknown killer. Several days after the crime, Speck tried to commit suicide by slashing his wrists and was brought to County. This was a full decade before my time at County, but the story of his capture there was legendary. An orthopedic intern cleaning off the blood from the man's self-inflicted wounds noticed a tattoo on his arm reading BORN TO RAISE HELL, matching the description given by the one surviving victim. The orthopedic intern notified the police and briefly became a national hero.

I took care of a couple of other slightly less notorious killers, one who stalked and killed people on the interstate and another who committed the heinous crime of killing her child. The latter patient also had an unforget-table stare.

Some famous non-criminals, such as down-and-out former celebrities, were also forced by circumstances to come to County Hospital. It was obvious why: they had fallen on hard times and were now charity cases.

One of my patients was a well-known rhythm and blues singer. He had several hit records, including a number one on the R&B charts in the mid-1960s. Several of his hits made the top twenty on the Billboard 100; they're still played on oldies stations today. Thirty years later, by the time I took care of him, his career had been wrecked by fast living and questionable management. His voice, looks, and whatever money he had made—everything that hadn't been gobbled up by managers and record labels—were gone, but he was still a good-natured guy with many great stories about working with singers like Jackie Wilson and Curtis Mayfield. He died long ago, but when I happen to hear one of his songs on the radio, I think of him fondly.

It wasn't unusual for former stars of baseball's Negro leagues, from the days before Jackie Robinson and the integration of the sport, to get their care at County Hospital. None of these patients were well known, but they had known and played against the immortals. They all had their own stories of Josh Gibson, Cool Papa Bell, and of course Satchel Paige. One patient, in his eighties, had been a longtime catcher in the Negro leagues. I asked him if he'd ever caught Satchel Paige. He smiled and held up his hand. Three of his fingers were gnarled and disfigured.

"Catching Satchel Paige did that."

I also took care of the father of a man who was, for a time in the 1970s, among the most popular people in the world. The famous son was the instantly recognizable star of a popular 1970s television sitcom, costar of several major motion pictures, and was frequently on the cover of *People* magazine. He certainly made quite a stir when he came to the ward to visit his father. The staff wondered why the son did not take his father to a more prestigious hospital. I didn't know, and never asked, but I like to think he was there by choice because of the quality of our care.

One of the most memorable celebrity stories I heard at County Hospital was about a movie star who had died decades before. A morgue attendant told it to me. Located in the basement of the old hospital, the morgue was unimaginably creepy. There were unclaimed bodies, corpses waiting for autopsies, and victims of foul play for whom the police were still working to solve the crime. It was set far away from the rest of the hospital, and most people had no reason to visit the place.

There were all kinds of grisly stories about the County morgue, many of which I'm sure were apocryphal. One of the best stories was written by Ben Hecht, the talented Chicago journalist and writer who eventually moved to New York to become a playwright and then to Hollywood to work as a prominent screenwriter. (He was the author of *The Front Page*, which also became the model for the movie *His Girl Friday*.) Before all this, Hecht wrote a short story about an early-twentieth-century Chicago police sergeant. The character describes what the morgue might have been like in the days right after World War I:

> I remember one night out to the old morgue. This was 'way back when I started on the force thirty years ago and more. And they was having trouble at the morgue owing to the stiffs vanishing and being mutilated. They thought maybe it was students carryin' them off to practice medicine on. But it wasn't, because they found old Pete—that was the colored janitor they had out there—he wasn't an African, but it turned out a Fiji Islander afterward. They found him dead in the morgue one day and it turned out he was a cannibal in Fiji, and the old habit had come up in him so he couldn't help himself, and he was makin' a diet off the bodies in the morgue. But he struck one that was embalmed, and the poison in the

body killed him. The papers didn't carry much on it on account of it not bein' very important, but I always thought it was kind of interestin' at that.

I don't know if that story was true, or whether Ben Hecht knew if it was true. But having visited the morgue, I can say it could have been true. The morgue was that chilling.

I would have to visit the morgue occasionally to check the status of the autopsy on a patient we'd taken care of. If we wanted to know the cause of death and the family agreed to a postmortem exam, the body would be held in the morgue until the pathologists could do the autopsy. A visit there was eerie, but somehow *eerie* doesn't do the place complete justice. The lighting was always dim enough that you had to strain your eyes to see across the room. Because it was located in the basement, and the bodies had to be kept cold, the temperature there was always around fifty degrees. It always felt chilly down there, winter or summer. There was a large floor scale that you had to step on to enter the room. It was always set at three hundred pounds below the zero line. When I asked the morgue attendant why, he said it was because the wheel-cart that transported bodies weighed exactly three hundred pounds, so they just subtracted that to figure out a body's weight. I made a point of checking my weight every time I went down there, and the closer I got to zero, the more it provided a morbid reminder that I had to lose a little weight.

For years, the morgue attendant was the same guy each time I went down there. He had apparently held the position for decades. *Straight out of central casting.* Short and stooped over, not old but not young. His grin was frozen like that of the Joker, and he had a limp like Igor from the Frankenstein movies. He wore a rumpled, dirty lab coat that reeked of formaldehyde.

I visited the morgue often enough that he came to know me. I occasionally brought residents with me, and none of them ever returned for a second visit. I was told that even the cops didn't like to go there.

Once I was checking on an autopsy, and after the attendant opened a locker to remove the body, I asked him, "Did you ever have anybody famous down here?"

I was figuring he might tell me about some second-level holdover hoodlum from the Capone era. But the morgue attendant became more animated than I had ever seen him. The pallor in his face disappeared momentarily.

"Are you kidding me? Do you know who I had down here? LINDA DARNELL. LINDA DARNELL. *I had Linda Darnell, in one of those lockers right over there.* They brought her in from the burn unit. She might have been good-looking when she was a big star, but she wasn't much to look at when I got her. That's right. Linda Darnell."

He kept repeating her name and he seemed to be in a hypnotic trance as he recalled her. It made the residents with me so uncomfortable that I got everyone out of there quickly.

Of course, none of the residents had any idea who Linda Darnell was. While I had a vague recollection of her being a glamorous movie star from an earlier era, I didn't know why the attendant was so exercised. I was curious. Was he just babbling about some long-ago fixation on a movie star? Was he even telling the truth? Was Linda Darnell even dead and if she was, what would she have been doing in the County morgue in Chicago? That night, I decided to look up details about Linda Darnell.

It turned out she was one of Hollywood's glamour girls in the early 1940s. She had a beautiful face and a figure to match. While she was still in her early twenties, she starred opposite Tyrone Power in *The Mark of Zorro* and *Blood and Sand*, and then opposite Henry Fonda in *My Darling Clementine*. For a short time, she was a huge box office star.

She wasn't a bad actress, but got by more on her looks than her acting. After the war, Hollywood, as it is wont to do, gradually replaced her with a bevy of younger glamour girls. Her acting could not carry her movie career and the roles became fewer and farther between. By the 1960s, she was basically out of movies, and in the spring of 1965 she was doing dinner theater in the northern suburbs of Chicago. Quite a comedown for a lady who was once one of Hollywood's biggest stars.

She was staying at the house of her former secretary, watching an old movie on television that she had starred in when she was only seventeen. It was about a girl who gets a Hollywood contract but then is turned down because she is too young—which is exactly what happened to Linda in real life. Who knows what this middle-aged woman, once the toast of Hollywood, thought when she watched her young self on the screen that night?

It was the last movie she ever saw.

A fire broke out and she was trapped in the house. She was alive when the firemen arrived, but she was badly burned over most of her body. She was taken to a small suburban hospital but quickly transferred to the County Burn Unit, at that time one of the best in the country. She died there the next day, only forty-one years old, a famous Hollywood star less than two decades removed from the height of her career. Before going to California for burial, her body must have been taken down to the basement and placed in the locker the morgue attendant had pointed to.

So he was probably telling the truth. By my reckoning, when that attendant was a young man in 1940, he probably went to *The Mark of Zorro* or *My Darling Clementine* and ogled one of Hollywood's most beautiful women and biggest stars. He would've had no idea of the macabre circumstances in which he would meet her twenty-five years later. Just like Richard Speck and me, when I was delivering newspapers with Speck's crime in the headlines.

To this day, I seek out old Linda Darnell movies at night on television. On the small screen in black-and-white, she is invariably beautiful and enchanting. But every time I see her, the sights and sounds of the County morgue come to mind, and I can never quite get them out.

19

TALES FROM THE MOVIES

"All right, Mr. DeMille, I'm ready for my close-up."
— NORMA DESMOND, *SUNSET BOULEVARD* (1950)

MOVIES OR TELEVISION shows about doctors or hospitals usually need a technical adviser to ensure that the medical details are accurate. Physicians frequently perform this role for the directors and showrunners. Even so, it's surprising how often the medical aspects don't come out right in the finished product. I got my chance to be a technical adviser once, and I'm proud to say that, with certain allowances, the medical details of the film I worked on were pretty accurate. Whether the movie is good or bad, that's your goal as a technical adviser.

The film was the 1993 thriller *The Fugitive*, starring Harrison Ford. As technical adviser, I worked with Ford as he developed his character, Dr. Richard Kimble. He is an excellent actor and his performance is brilliant; in all modesty, he did put just a little bit of me there in his screen portrayal. Most people have a fantasy of who would best play them in a movie, and for me, this was the closest I will ever come to being portrayed on the big screen. It's certainly possible the lede for my obituary will read, "Model for Harrison Ford's character in *The Fugitive*." I'm fortunate the actor I worked for happened to be one of the best of our generation. Made my technical work look better.

It's an unusual opportunity to be part of a major Hollywood movie, and while you don't get paid much, you do come away with lots of stories about celebrities and the movie industry. My involvement started when I got a call from the director, a Chicago South Sider and great guy named Andy Davis. He started out directing in Chicago in the 1970s. I first ran into him years before *The Fugitive*, at a 1978 showing of a small local indie film he directed about Chicago jazz musicians. The movie, *Stony Island*, was acclaimed by the critics but bombed at the box office. It had a minor renaissance when it was rereleased on DVD in 2012.

Despite the commercial failure of *Stony Island*, Andy left for Hollywood and became hugely successful, especially after directing the Steven Seagal blockbuster *Under Siege*. On the heels of that, Warner Bros. selected him to make *The Fugitive*. The story was a loose adaptation of the popular 1960s television show, which in turn loosely paralleled the 1954 Sam Sheppard murder case in Ohio (although the creators of the television series, perhaps for legal reasons, deny they based the show on the actual case). Warner gave him a $40 million budget for the movie and they managed to sign Harrison Ford to be the box office draw.

To make the movie, Davis decided to come back to his hometown, Chicago. Apparently, when he was looking for a technical adviser for the medical aspects of the movie, several people recommended me. When Andy came to town, he called me and asked if I would like to work on the movie. He said he remembered meeting me and told me I came highly recommended. He said he needed someone to work with his star on how to be a doctor. I did not remember meeting him fifteen years before, so the whole thing seemed out of the blue to me. The next thing he said was that he would arrange for Harrison Ford to meet me in my office the next Wednesday; Ford was coming to have me teach him to play a doctor.

Talking to a movie director is not part of your average day in the hospital. An hour before, this was not even on my radar. I had no inkling what was coming. Now, not only would I be working on a movie, but a Hollywood actor who was perhaps the biggest star in the world would be coming to see me. By 1992, Ford had starred in what were then seven of the twenty-five highest-grossing films of all time: three films from the *Indiana Jones* series, three from the *Star Wars* series, and *American Graffiti*. His films had grossed far in excess of $1 billion. More than two decades later, he remains one of the highest-grossing actors in history.

Our meeting was still a week away and I still wasn't sure all this was really going to happen, so I put it out of my mind. By the following Wednesday, I had actually forgotten all about it. I was coming back to my office after lunch and something was clearly going on. There was a line of nurses at my secretary's desk about half a block long. I asked the secretary what was up.

He said, "Which story do you want? The made-up story or the real one?"

I still didn't get it. He explained, "The cover story is that the copy machine in your office is the only one in the building that's working. But the real reason the nurses are here is that Harrison Ford is sitting in your office and they want to get a glimpse of him"

It was true. I summarily dispersed the nurses and walked into my office, and there an informally dressed man introduced himself to me: "Harrison Ford."

You don't get many moments like that. What do you say?

I just introduced myself, and he simply said, "I'll be working with you."

He didn't stay very long. I showed him around the ICU, and took him on a brief tour of the hospital, during which everyone stopped to stare at him. I was uneasy, but I sensed that he was quite used to it and paid them no mind.

It reminded me of a story I had heard about Albert Einstein accompanying Charlie Chaplin to one of the silent comedian's film premieres. Einstein got into Chaplin's limousine, and as they neared the theater, the crowd swelled around the car to get a look at Chaplin, then the most famous man in the world. As the crowd swarmed dangerously close to the car, Einstein, unfamiliar with this degree of adulation, grew visibly afraid. He turned to Chaplin, who did not seem at all interested or concerned about the mob, no doubt because it had all become routine to him.

A frightened Einstein asked, "What does all this mean?"

Chaplin, without showing any emotion, said simply, "Nothing. Nothing at all."

Ford was like that. He asked very few questions. I later realized that he was trying to make me comfortable, the better to help him do his job. One of the first things I learned was that good actors are superb students of human behavior. I have known some doctors who were pretty good at studying people, but Harrison Ford was better than any of them. He knew I would be uncomfortable with people fawning over him, and he was right. Without saying anything, he was reassuring me, letting me know that he was quite serious about learning what I could teach him. He shook my hand and left quickly.

A nice guy, all business, and a true professional. Once my wife asked me if she could invite him to dinner. I never broached the subject with him. In fact, I never even asked him for his autograph. I regret that now; I probably should have, so I would have some token of the experience, but it would have seemed unnatural when we were working together.

The next day, I received a call from one of the Hollywood assistants. I was to meet Mr. Davis, Mr. Ford, and the screenwriters that night at a posh and extremely expensive Michigan Avenue restaurant, one that I would never go to unless someone else was paying. When I later met that Hollywood assistant, he was wearing an open shirt and gold chains, and carrying a big brick cell phone, circa 1992. Some stereotypes turn out to be true.

I got to the restaurant early, and when Ford walked in everyone gawked at him. Our table was blocked off from the other customers and the maître d' gave strict orders to the waiters that we were not to be disturbed. The dinner conversation was a mixture of business, movies, medicine, and informal banter. I would have remained silent, but the screenwriters peppered me with questions. They had the basic structure of the movie—doctor wrongly convicted of killing his wife escapes from prison to search for the real killer—but they needed medical details to fill in the plot. Ford said very little, but once again I realized later that he was studying very closely what I said and how I said it.

It got annoying with waiters fawning about incessantly, but for the Hollywood people it was apparently nothing unusual. It really is a different world.

When we discussed medicine, I mentioned the medical school lecture I had given that afternoon about drug companies, doctors, and the conflicts of interest doctors face. I explained how pharmaceutical companies offered conference junkets to doctors as an indirect means of bribing them. The screenwriters were quite intrigued by this, and when I told them the medical school made a video of my lecture, they were excited to see it. I didn't know they would skillfully weave these ideas into the story.

(In the film, Kimble's wife is murdered because the good doctor's work poses a threat to some nefarious pharmaceutical firm. It was originally supposed to be a more important part of the story, but Richard Jordan, the actor who was to play one of the villains, died during the filming. Because of this, the story had to be modified, but the pharmaceutical junket is still central to the movie.)

At one point, the screenwriters asked me about medical terms, and how doctors talk and react to different situations. One turned to me and said, "Tell us something that people say to you all the time. You know, at parties or something."

I gave it a minute's thought and said offhandedly, "You know, at parties people come up to me and they always say, 'I should have been a doctor.' Lots of people out there think they should have been doctors."

Six months later, I watched a preview showing of the movie with an audience of people who had worked on the set. About halfway through the film, Tommy Lee Jones, who plays Inspector Sam Gerard, the man looking for Richard Kimble, puts down a medical brochure and says to his officers, *"I should have been a doctor."*

When I saw that in the theater the first time, I thought to myself, "Hey, that's my line!" It's exhilarating to hear a chunk of dialogue you added to the movie. You have to keep yourself from "going Hollywood." But I decided no open shirt, gold chains, and big brick cell phone for me.

───────────

Despite the popular conception, making movies is not the business Hollywood is in. The real business of Hollywood is understanding people's reactions and emotions, and learning how to manipulate them. Movies are simply the vehicle for doing that, and the best films and actors are the ones most skillful at manipulation. Billions of dollars change hands every year on the strength of successfully manipulating people's reactions and emotions.

I witnessed this when the director wanted my wife to be an extra in the film. There was a banquet scene at the Four Seasons and they needed extras to fill the banquet room. As director, Andy Davis liked to put friends, relatives, and local people into background scenes and nonspeaking roles. So that same Hollywood assistant, Mr. Open Shirt, asked me for our home phone number so he could pitch my wife about being an extra. I gave the number to him, but told him my wife was shy and would probably refuse to be in the movie. He called her at home anyway, early in the morning.

Mr. Open Shirt had never met my wife and did not know her from Adam. Nevertheless, this did not prevent him from immediately calling her by her first name when she answered the phone. Another stereotype that turned out to be true: Hollywood assistants like addressing people they don't know by their first names.

"Sue?"

"Who is this?"

"I'm working on *The Fugitive* with Cory."

"Is he all right?" (My wife worries a lot.)

"He's fine. The reason I'm calling is we want you to be in the movie."

"What?"

"As an extra. We have a crowd scene at the Four Seasons downtown, and we'd like you to be one of the people in the large banquet room. You wouldn't have to do anything."

"Thank you, but I don't think so."

It was just as I had told him. But as I said, these people are experts at understanding reactions and manipulating them.

"Look, Sue, I understand how you feel. We will let you bring a friend to be with you as an extra. Look at it this way. It will be a once in a lifetime opportunity and you can share it with a friend."

Think about the manipulation. How many people are going to say no, when it is posed to them like that? My wife agreed reluctantly, brought a friend, and spent a day being an extra. I'm pretty sure she was left on the cutting room floor, but I think her friend's backside made it into the crowd scene.

————————

When I worked with Harrison Ford, he was studying me, but I also couldn't help noticing things about him and the people around him. Once I had a cafeteria lunch with a young actress who played an emergency room doctor in the movie. She was a beautiful redhead, quite pleasant, unpretentious, and witty. Today, she is an Academy Award–winning star: Julianne Moore. At lunch, I was not surprised when she confessed to having something of a schoolgirl crush on Harrison Ford. Understandable. Most of the women who came in contact with him, like those nurses in line outside my office, felt the same way.

Actors treat fellow actors differently from the way other people treat them. I observed that most non-actors on the movie set were quite deferential to Ford—sometimes, in my opinion, overly so. People were always bowing and scraping in front of him, and while he never gave any indication that he noticed, surely he did. However, I quickly understood that this was the natural reaction to being around him; in fact, it was the *expected* reaction. Some sort of etiquette dictated that you weren't supposed to get too familiar with him. I did have lunch in director Andy Davis's trailer, but I was *never* allowed in the inner sanctum of Harrison Ford's trailer. It would have been out of the question.

This issue of how to behave while working with a major actor put me in an uncomfortable position. I didn't want to act like a sycophant, even if it was expected. Neither could I be too aloof. No one liked that attitude, especially from a lowly technical adviser.

My role seemed to shift once the movie was in production. Before filming started, when the Hollywood people were persuading me to come on board the project, they kept telling me I was the only doctor they would trust with this assignment. They were, of course, playing on my vanity—and it worked. However, the moment I was committed, their attitude changed. It was not subtle in any way: "Just do what we say and don't give us any trouble," they said. "There are five hundred guys out there who can do what you are doing, and we are ready to get them on a moment's notice."

So my dilemma when working with Harrison Ford was, how do I behave? I imagine a lot of people are faced with this problem when they are around celebrities or important people. Fawning flattery or cool indifference?

Why not just be yourself?

Ultimately that is what I settled on, but it's not as easy as it sounds. When everyone around you is groveling, it's hard not to grovel yourself.

And if you come off as too distant, you can be summarily fired. After all, as they told me, there were plenty of others who could do the job.

One day on the set, the director was filming a scene of people walking down a hospital hallway. He wanted my secretary and me to be two of the extras in the scene. I demurred, telling him I'm not a camera guy, but to no avail. Both of us were enlisted as extras. We walked down the hallway about twenty times; two hours shooting for a fifteen-second scene.

Around the second hour of shooting, Harrison Ford wandered on the set to watch. He obviously enjoyed seeing us struggling through shot after shot. Like a professional golfer watching a couple of duffers. All we had to do was walk, no dialogue, but we had no idea what we were doing, and whether what we were doing was causing all the reshoots. Ford sat there, drinking a cup of coffee, chuckling to himself at the amateurs screwing up. Finally, they called a break and Ford motioned to me to come over.

He offered me a cup of coffee and a seat next to him. Then he said, facetiously, "You were terrific out there."

I borrowed that line from *Sunset Boulevard*: "I take it I'm not ready for my close-up with Mr. DeMille."

He laughed, "No, not yet."

Then we sat there drinking coffee for a few minutes. Neither of us said anything, and it was one of those situations where the silence became uncomfortable. I'm sitting next to the biggest box office star in the world and I don't know what to say. The thought flashed through my mind: *Fawning flattery or cool indifference?*

I didn't want to say anything stupid or servile, but continued silence next to a famous Hollywood star might be interpreted as cool indifference. I felt I was expected to say something to break the silence. But what could I say?

Just be yourself.

My mind raced. What might I say to one of my friends in that situation? I would probably talk about work or current events. As it happened, it was the night of the Academy Awards. He wasn't nominated or involved, but

I figured it would be a good topic to break the silence. After all, he surely knew everyone who was nominated. So I thought I would ask.

"So, give me your professional opinion. Who do you think is going to win at the Oscars tonight?"

I should have known better. He was not an awards type of person. He gave me a withering look and said, "I really couldn't care less about any of that stuff. I mean, really, who cares?"

That struck me as sort of a blasé answer. But here's where it is hard to be yourself. Had one of my friends said something like that, I probably would have replied sarcastically, "Excuse me, Mr. Big Shot."

That would have been the "just be yourself" answer. But I never gave a thought to saying that. Instead, I agreed with him. "Right, right, all that Oscar stuff is superficial crap."

He nodded and went back to his trailer. No matter how hard I had tried, I ultimately reverted to fawning sycophancy. And our "walking down the hall" scene never made it into the movie. That's show business.

———————

When Hollywood calls, it's a good idea to answer only when asked. One of my jobs as technical adviser was to make sure the medical set always looked as realistic as possible. Some of the filming was done in a refurbished three-story school building on the South Side. One floor of the school was made to look like a prison (where the convict Richard Kimble is sent), another floor was made to resemble a prosthetics lab, and one floor was supposed to be a hospital emergency area. That last floor was my responsibility.

One day, some of Mr. Open Shirt's underlings brought me to the emergency room set. There were extras wandering around dressed as doctors, nurses, security guards, janitors, etc. My charge was to guarantee verisimilitude in the physical details.

It was fun walking around giving suggestions to make a movie set look like a hospital ward. There was a blank whiteboard on a wall, and I had to create a fictional nursing shift assignment, complete with made-up patients' names, nurses' names, and room numbers. (Today, HIPAA, the Health Insurance Portability and Accountability Act, would prohibit what was once considered routine procedure.)

My word carried weight. When I was asked what books might be found at the nurses' station, I replied we needed a nursing handbook and a *Physicians' Desk Reference*, the encyclopedic medication manual all hospitals rely on. Some assistant snapped his finger and some lower-level assistant was sent out to get them. A couple of hours later, those books were on the ward.

When I was done furnishing the emergency room, it looked pretty good. Between the medical details and the realistic-looking cast, you might really believe you were in a hospital. Then I learned another lesson about Hollywood.

Show business wants reality, just not too much of it.

The next day I came to the set to watch the shooting. It was a simple scene, a bunch of extras dressed as hospital personnel and patients walking down the hallway. I received several compliments on how realistic the background looked. They told me I did a good job and I should feel really proud—and I did. As they shot the scene, I felt as though I was really part of the movie.

Until about the third take, when an actor suddenly came rollerblading down the hall. I think he was supposed to be an orderly. While he was only on camera for about five seconds, I was struck by the incongruity of someone rollerblading in the hospital. In my mind, it destroyed the realism of the scene.

By then, I was feeling pretty confident, even cocky. After all, I'd just helped put all this together. So at that point, I went to the person in charge of the scene and said, "You know, that would never happen in a real hospital. Nobody rollerblades down the hall."

Wrong thing to say. I'd forgotten their admonition: "Just do what we say and don't give us any trouble." The assistant director, or whoever he was, gave me a cold stare. At that moment, all my past contributions to the movie didn't mean anything. He immediately let me know where I really stood in the hierarchy: "When we want your opinion, we will ask for it. Got that?"

The rollerblading orderly stayed in the movie, and I very nearly didn't.

———————

Sometimes, as Orson Welles's character is told in *Citizen Kane*, "You're going to need more than one lesson, and you're going to get more than one lesson." Unfortunately, I heard the line "When we want your opinion, we will ask for it. Got that?" once more before the end of the movie.

Harrison Ford and I were working together on a scene that I really enjoyed. The plot point was that Dr. Kimble is undercover in the hospital as a janitor when they bring a young boy to the emergency room with chest trauma. The little boy is supposed to have a life-threatening condition, a tension pneumothorax, which will be immediately evident on his chest X-ray. Once diagnosed, the little boy will have to go to surgery.

As Kimble, the janitor who was really a doctor, observes the situation, he sees the doctor who is taking care of the patient leave him without looking at the X-ray. Julianne Moore, the head doctor, tells the "janitor" to move the patient to an examining room, but instead Kimble looks at the X-ray, makes the diagnosis, and diverts the patient to the operating room and the surgery that will eventually save the little boy's life.

While Ford and I were discussing the scene, he asked me what I would do at every point in the situation. He was especially curious about how I would act as I wheeled the boy into the elevator to go to the operating room. It wasn't completely scripted, so what should he say?

I told him, "The first thing you have to remember is that the little boy will be afraid. He is in a strange situation, he is having trouble breathing, he has severe chest pain, and he is really scared. What you want to do is take his fear away. Reassure him. He wants to know where his mother is. Tell him she's coming. And then what I would do is talk to him about something else he's interested in that takes his mind off the current situation. Ask him if he plays sports. Baseball, football, whatever. Assure him everything is going to be OK.

Let me tell you, Harrison Ford did that elevator ride with the kid better than I would have. In fact, about as well as anyone could do it. Olivier, Brando, De Niro—nobody could have reassured that kid better than he did. He was so good, I thought they should use that segment to teach doctors how to talk to frightened children. He could be a technical adviser to doctors. I watched the scene that day with Andy Davis and we were both ecstatic about how it came off. So much so, that we decided to watch it again together.

And then I saw the mistake: *the perfect is the enemy of the good.*

The second time we watched it, I noticed one of those movie gaffes that every movie has. As Ford wheels the young boy into the elevator, he looks at the X-ray.

And he is looking at it backwards.

Now, this is not really a big deal, and the shot lasts for less than five seconds. But when your job is technical accuracy, you are supposed to notice things like that. So I felt compelled to say something to the director. Of course, it never occurred to me that reshooting the whole scene just for that minor error would be a significant undertaking, and there was no guarantee it would come off as smoothly as it did the first time. So I said to Andy, "Andy, watch right there. Kimble is looking at the X-ray backward. The heart is on the right, but it's supposed to be on the left. Any doctor would flip it around to look at it."

It took me longer to say that than it had taken Ford to look at the X-ray.

Davis looked at me sternly and said, just about verbatim from the way the other guy had said it before, "When we want your opinion we will ask for it."

I got it. From then on, it was speak only when spoken to.

It's funny, but until the shooting was over, I had no idea what I would be paid. When I'd signed on to work on the movie, Andy Davis and I never talked about money. It would have been unseemly. The unstated assump-tion was that I was lucky to get this chance. They knew I was unlikely to ask—remember, their business is knowing how people will react.

It's a great movie. It was nominated for Best Picture of 1993 (though the Academy Award went to *Schindler's List*). The movie grossed over $350 million worldwide in theaters, and tens of millions more in video rentals and who knows what else. Maybe it ultimately made half a billion. And in the end, I got $1,100.

Next time, I'll hire an agent.

20

STAY AWAY FROM THE HOSPITAL ON HOLIDAYS IF AT ALL POSSIBLE

"'Twas the night before Christmas and all through the house,
not a creature was stirring . . . nothin' . . . no action . . . dullsville!"

—Margie MacDougall, *The Apartment* (1960)

THE BRILLIANT FILM director Billy Wilder loved to use holidays as a recurring theme in his most memorable movies. Christmas was a key setting in *Stalag 17* and *The Apartment*. New Year's Eve was an essential element of *The Apartment* and *Sunset Boulevard*. And Yom Kippur, the Jewish Day of Atonement, was central to the plot of *The Lost Weekend*. Wilder, more than any other film director, knew intuitively that there was drama and a special emotional pull when he placed his characters in holiday settings.

Those same elements of drama and emotional pull—abounding with both joy and sadness—are at work in the hospital on the major holidays.

All hospitals, even the best ones, are more lightly staffed on holidays. Critical areas like the emergency department, trauma, and intensive care usually have relatively consistent nursing coverage regardless of holidays. But general wards often have fewer nurses on duty, and for major holidays, ancillary personnel like therapists and secretaries have the day off. Those who do have to work sometimes cross-cover, staffing areas that are less familiar to them. Senior administrative personnel usually have the day off, leaving junior administrators to deal with problems.

Physician coverage is also different on major holidays. Some physicians come in on holidays to make rounds; other doctors take calls at home. Where I worked it was common for doctors to do religious swapping: observant Jewish doctors would do rounds on Christmas and Easter in exchange for having their non-Jewish counterparts do rounds on Jewish holidays.

In hospitals that employ residents, junior residents are generally the primary workforce on major holidays. Many specialists, particularly those less likely to be needed in emergencies, take the day off; consultations with certain specialists may be postponed. If not, they are done by doctors unfamiliar with the patient or by less experienced junior doctors. Radiology and respiratory or physical therapy might be staffed lightly, depending on the patient population. If a patient happened to need a particular specialist, unless it was an emergency, the specialist might hear about the case by phone and then see the patient the next day. Lots of specialists have a busy Friday the day after Thanksgiving.

On holidays, staff camaraderie tends to be greater, probably because of a shared sense of misery over having to work when others have the day off. It's not unusual to see hospital workers share holiday gestures with coworkers, patients, and families—like having a brief midnight celebration on New Year's Eve, sharing a special meal on Thanksgiving, or bringing small gifts on Christmas. Some nurse is likely to have a Santa hat on, or at the very least a set of reindeer antlers.

In the general wards of the hospital, the difference in staffing can be more pronounced and more problematic. All things being equal, I have always counseled patients to avoid scheduling elective surgery and admissions around Memorial Day, Labor Day, Thanksgiving, Christmas, and

New Year's Eve, if at all possible. Even for minor surgeries it's better to have a complete staff on duty.

(Interestingly, the problem of holiday coverage is not confined to the United States. In Pakistan, patients have problems when doctors and medical staff take off during the Muslim holiday of Eid, at the end of Ramadan. One newspaper quoted an attendant at the Lahore Services Hospital: "Nobody is there to listen to the grievances of patients or their attendants because the entire administration of the hospital is enjoying holidays." The newspaper reported that other major Pakistani hospitals including Lahore General Hospital, Jinnah Hospital, and Sir Ganga Ram Hospital experienced a lack of diagnostic services during this time.)

Because most American hospitals begin their training schedules for new residents on July 1, the Independence Day holiday is a special case. In their first week of formal training, residents are sent out to work in an environment with less staffing and fewer specialists. Most good hospitals are aware of this potential problem and provide extra coverage accordingly.

A frequently circulated urban myth is that July is the worst time to be sick, because of the inexperience of the staff. Studies have examined this, and most of them refute this theory; mortality is not consistently higher that month. In my hospital's department of medicine, I studied data from nearly three decades, and there was no increase in mortality in July. Ironically, some observers theorize that August, not July, may actually be a more dangerous month, since at that point inexperienced doctors are on their own more often, no longer backed by extra coverage. Still others have postulated June as the most dangerous month, because so many resident doctors are graduating at the end of the month and therefore might have a tendency to slack off, experiencing the med school equivalent of "senioritis." There is little evidence to support those theories either.

It is more likely, in fact, that physician experience is only a minor factor in determining hospital outcomes. Hospital mortality rates are affected far more significantly by *case mix*, the types of diseases and patients that characterize the hospital population. In northern climes, mortality may be higher in the winter, when there are far more communicable respiratory problems like pneumonia and influenza, than in the summer, when new physicians have less experience. At least at our hospital, the Christmas season was a more dangerous time than July 4—with the exception of the summer of 1995, when mortality soared due to a historic summer heat wave that became a major cardiovascular stressor.

Elsewhere, especially in hospitals where surgeons take care of trauma, there is often a higher mortality rate in the summer, almost certainly due to the increases in blunt and penetrating injuries that occur in the summer months. More people are outside, and that brings a concomitant increase in motor vehicle accidents, as well as in crimes such as shootings or stabbings that result in serious injury. For surgical patients, July is generally a dangerous time regardless of the surgeon's level of experience. Sometimes even the most practiced surgeon can't put Humpty Dumpty with multiple injuries back together again.

Holidays also change the composition of patients entering the emergency room. Most people understandably put off the routine problems that would ordinarily send them to the hospital. One ER-experienced doctor I know was adamant that the slowest evening of the year in the ER was that all-American holiday Super Bowl Sunday. Perhaps, but I have seen no evidence to confirm it. What doctors do tend to see on holidays is what you'd expect: carving and cooking mishaps during holiday feasts, or injuries from outdoor activities in summertime. Expect firecracker injuries on July 4, serious scald burns on Thanksgiving and Christmas, and an increase in drunk driving accidents on New Year's. Several studies have noted a greater incidence of depression during the holidays, so there may also be an increase in suicide attempts. And of course, at every holiday there are alcohol-related problems—lots of them.

I heard a fascinating story from a person who works with organ donation. Transplant candidates often get their organs from victims of car accidents. Since there are more fatal crashes during holidays, some potential recipients have admitted experiencing a subtle stirring of morbid hope during the holidays that an organ donor will emerge from a car crash. (According to the National Highway Traffic Safety Administration, the five most dangerous holidays for drivers are, in order, Thanksgiving, July 4, Memorial Day weekend, Labor Day weekend, and New Year's Eve/Day.)

However abstract it seems, organ recipients know that somewhere out there on Thanksgiving weekend a motorcyclist going too fast or a car-versus-tree collision will result in a heart, kidney, or liver donation. The flip side is that once the holiday is over and the donor has not received a call, he or she may become depressed over the lost opportunity. I know of no studies to confirm this, but there is a certain perverse logic to it.

A longtime colleague told me a poignant story about his experience in the hospital during Christmas. One year, he drew the assignment to be the anesthesiologist working for the operating room in case there were any surgical emergencies on Christmas Day. It was a slow day; there wasn't a single case. So everyone—the surgical team, nursing staff, and orderlies—sat around the lounge playing Monopoly. From his description, I imagined lots of Santa hats and reindeer antlers on people who would much rather have been with their families, and perhaps an uneaten fruitcake on the table next to the Monopoly board.

Twenty-five years later, he still remembers it vividly. And as he confided with a sly wink, "That day I learned the true meaning of Christmas: buying Boardwalk and Park Place."

21

YES, PHYSICIANS CAN BE ARROGANT AND HEARTLESS

"To be faithful to that trust, the physician must avoid the vice of arrogance, one of the most frequent complaints I hear from patients. The inequality of power and knowledge between doctors and patients feeds the inordinate pride and self-importance that most physicians exhibit at one time or another."

—DR. EDMUND PELLEGRINO

SURVEYS SUGGEST THAT many people don't like doctors in general, but they tend to like *their* doctor. Among the criticisms patients voice about doctors is that some are arrogant and others are cold. This aspect of the medical profession is touched on more in fiction than nonfiction; it is a common plotline in movies and novels. Most nonfiction accounts of physician arrogance or heartlessness tend to be written by patients who have had bad experiences. More often, doctors who are authors avoid the subject of egregious physician egotism. Ironically, some of the worst physician behavior occurs in conferences and meetings, where no one is there to observe it but other physicians. I saw it many times, and in two cases I spoke up, perhaps when I should not have. In both cases, my arch remarks were punished summarily.

During my residency, when I worked on a medical service, we would have a daily morning report and discuss cases before the chief of medicine in his office. On Saturdays everything was less formal, and on this particular Saturday the medicine chief, a product of the counterculture of the 1960s, decided the residents should sit in a circle on the floor while the previous night's pulmonary cases were presented. To reinforce their authority over us, neither the chief nor the top pulmonary attending sat on the floor.

One resident presented the case of a patient with tuberculosis of the lungs and failure of the adrenal glands. Occasionally, the tuberculosis bacillus attacks both organs, so it was an interesting case for discussion, especially in the informal setting. Most of the doctors there were sharp, well read, and intellectually curious. The discussion went back and forth for about fifteen minutes. Then the pulmonary attending, by his own account the world's foremost authority on tuberculosis, weighed in on the case.

The pulmonary attending was a tall, ostentatious man with a booming voice and a commanding presence. He was considered a blowhard by most of the residents, because he loved to shock his audience with his pronouncements, which were often ridiculous. As he towered over the residents sitting on the floor on this occasion, he didn't disappoint. He cut off the discussion of the case with a dramatic announcement that not only seemed to belie this particular case but also contradicted every medical textbook. He said imperiously, "There is no association between tuberculosis and failure of the adrenal glands."

This shocked everyone in the room, even the chief of medicine, who normally supported him. For a moment, everyone sat in stunned silence until the chief of medicine asked the logical follow-up question, "Dr. Masters, how can you say there is no association between tuberculosis and failure of the adrenal glands? It's reported in every textbook."

Undaunted, the pulmonary expert answered with a delivery John Barrymore in his prime would have envied: "There is no association because I have personally seen twelve hundred cases of tuberculosis and I have never seen a case of adrenal failure."

Pompous nonsense. Followed by more stunned silence. What to say to an authority figure who posits the ridiculous premise that because you have never seen something, it has never happened?

My resident colleagues turned to me, the wise-guy. With sarcasm dripping, I said, "Dr. Masters, have you ever seen a plane crash?"

He turned red, and I was immediately called out for my insubordination and banished from the room by the chief. My fellow residents, silently in support of my defiant remark, snickered to themselves as I left like a ballplayer who has just been ejected from the game.

My punishment was not yet complete. I was scheduled to do a special three-month rotation at a university hospital, during which County was supposed to pay my salary. When Dr. Masters heard about it, he went right to the chief of medicine and protested. The chief backed him up. I was allowed to do the rotation, but based on Dr. Masters's objections, County did not pay my salary. I worked for free for those three months. In those days a resident couldn't appeal that kind of thing. So that "plane crash" remark wound up costing me $10,000—a not inconsiderable sum, then or now.

I occasionally see a few colleagues who had been among the residents in the room that day. They are now respected, successful physicians, and every so often when we get together, we will relive that long-ago morning sitting on the floor. Surprisingly, some of them remember what had happened. They ask me if it was worth losing $10,000.

I always answer the same way Robert Redford did when Paul Newman asked him at the conclusion of *The Sting* if the con was worth it: "It's not enough. . . . But it's close."

From *Clinical Medicine & Research* (2008):

In 1855, Thomas Addison described autopsy findings of six patients with adrenal tuberculosis, which continues to be one of the most common causes of adrenal insufficiency in the developing world.

That was physician arrogance, but ironically it was on the next rotation, the unpaid one, that I encountered a worse combination: physician arrogance combined with utter heartlessness. Much of the best medicine practiced in America occurs in university hospitals. Not to denigrate rural and community hospitals, but if you are sick, especially with a rare disease, a university hospital is generally the best place to be. Nevertheless, the university hospital is among the most impersonal and occasionally arrogant institutions in America. Unfortunately, some doctors tend to emulate their surroundings.

On one of my last nights there, I was the senior resident on the resuscitation team, the group of four or five people who respond when the cardiac arrest beeper goes off. A junior resident in anesthesia, a brilliant young woman, was with me, and her job was to intubate the patient. That evening we were called to the emergency room, where a patient was brought in from the street in full cardiac arrest. The remainder of the team assembled quickly from their areas, and I was the team coordinator.

Everything has to go right for the resuscitation of a cardiac arrest victim to be successful. Even then, luck plays no small part. Quite often, there are either too many or too few people responding to a cardiac arrest. On television, you may see fifteen or even twenty doctors and nurses around the bed at a cardiac arrest. The best resuscitation procedures occur when there are between six and ten people responding. Any fewer and there is too much for each person to do; any more and chaos often ensues.

That night, including the emergency room staff and our team, we had nine people, just about the right number. During the resuscitation, things did go right, like a symphony perfectly played. Everyone did their jobs crisply and efficiently. In addition, fortune was on our side—and, more important, on the patient's side. Many victims of cardiac arrest do not survive, but in this case the junior resident intubated the patient quickly and the patient's heart responded to the defibrillator immediately. To bring someone back to life is among the most satisfying moments in the field of medicine.

The patient was immediately transported to the intensive care unit, where the ICU doctors and nurses took over his care. When a patient's heart stops, his brain loses oxygen. If the heart doesn't restart quickly, usually within five minutes, the patient suffers brain damage. We were otherwise not busy that night, so the junior resident and I were able to visit the ICU several times to check on the patient. By morning, he was awake and following commands. No brain damage. That made the night's efforts even more fulfilling.

At 8 AM, after a cup of coffee, the junior resident and I proceeded to our morning conference, where we had to review all our cases from the night before with the rest of the team and the senior attending. Despite the long evening, we felt invigorated; we had just saved a man's life. It was the junior resident's first successful resuscitation, and I let her present the case. She had earned that honor.

The senior attending was an expert in his field, well known throughout the country. He wrote books and gave lectures everywhere. He was also an arrogant, obnoxious man—even more so than Dr. Masters. During my time with him, he and I had jousted occasionally, but I generally tried to stay on his good side, because I needed a letter of recommendation. With his national reputation, his support would be invaluable for my future training.

Successful resuscitations being rare, I thought our performance the previous evening would go over well. It didn't. The junior resident began her presentation, "Mr. Taliaferro is a sixty-year-old white male who presented to the ER in full cardiac arrest . . ."

The attending did not know the outcome of the case and cut her off abruptly. Having experienced many unsuccessful resuscitations, the attending was pessimistic about the whole endeavor of trying to resuscitate people who had a cardiac arrest outside the hospital.

"Not another one of these. What a waste of time and money."

Several years before, he had been part of the team that was called to an out-of-hospital emergency when one of the country's most important public officials was in cardiac arrest. The resuscitation was unsuccessful and the patient died, because too much time had elapsed before the team could begin treatment. It was no fault of the doctor's, but I suspect he was somewhat bitter because, had he and the team been able to save the patient, they would have received national attention. I think that missed opportunity may have contributed to his cynicism about resuscitation efforts. I wondered what he would say when he heard about the outcome of this case.

The junior resident continued and described how the patient's heart was restarted. Still not impressed, the attending frowned and became more cynical. "So what? So you got his heart started again. Big deal. He'll probably be a vegetable. I've seen that too many times."

Again, he was unaware of how the story would end. His attitude left the resident so nonplussed, she could hardly continue. Here was a nationally known physician mocking her first successful resuscitation effort. In a barely audible voice, she explained that we had followed up on the patient in the ICU before the conference and the patient was alert and responding. He would not be a vegetable.

I watched the attending closely. Rather than congratulate us, as he should have done, he was scowling, because things had not turned out the way he expected. On an impulse, I challenged him because of his attitude. We had just saved a man's life and he blithely dismissed it.

Perhaps in retrospect, it was a mistake for me to say anything. After all, my smart mouth had already earned me three months without pay.

"Well, Dr. Schwartz, the patient survived and is neurologically intact. Maybe you should reevaluate your estimation of cardiac arrest resuscitation efforts in the emergency room."

His face displayed a barely concealed rage. His voice dropped, low and serious, and he gave me an icy stare. I had strayed into dangerous territory. He said, "Listen, it would have been no significant loss to humanity if this guy had died."

Everybody collectively gasped at such a callous remark. It was meant to silence the room.

This only increased my anger. By now I was in too deep. I couldn't let his remark pass. "Maybe you'd like to tell that to Mr. Taliaferro's wife and family."

Worse than the plane crash remark to Dr. Masters. And the consequences, while not as immediate, were even more devastating. He said nothing but gave me an even colder, harder stare.

About a week later, I came to his office to apologize. I had overstepped my bounds and I told him as much. He was unmoved. He probably believed my apology was done with the knowledge that I would need a letter of recommendation—and he was at least partly right. He accepted my apology perfunctorily. A month later, I came in to ask for a letter of recommendation. That's when he got his revenge.

When a junior physician requests a letter of recommendation from a prestigious doctor, the latter has several options. If he believes the candidate is good, he will write a nice letter. If he believes the candidate less so, he can write a letter in coded language that reveals his lack of enthusiasm to whomever the letter is intended for. In that respect, there are certain phrases in medical circles that are familiar as "damning with faint praise." By doing that, the doctor does not have to refuse the applicant's request. But on those occasions when the prestigious doctor believes a candidate is really bad, he can tell him politely that he is unable to write the letter.

Dr. Schwartz did none of those things. He agreed to my request and then, unbeknownst to me, he wrote a scathing letter. In his eyes, I was an incompetent who should never be allowed near patients.

Normally, I would never have known this, but I was rejected from a position I thought I was sure to get. I asked the physician responsible why

I didn't get the post, and he mailed me a copy of Dr. Schwartz's referral letter. He said that in his experience he had never seen a letter like it, which was probably true. I wound up at another postgraduate program, one that Dr. Schwartz did not send the letter to. He came close to ending my career with that letter.

Dr. Schwartz is long dead. Many years later, before he died, I saw him at a conference where he was one of the guest speakers. He gave me a friendly smile. Maybe he did not remember what had happened years before. I thanked him for his long-ago letter of recommendation and his smile widened.

I don't know what that cryptic smile meant. Maybe it meant he did remember what had happened years before. I will never know. There was then, and still is today, a lot of arrogance and callousness in medicine. It is generally not a good idea to challenge it directly. You can fight city hall, but you will probably lose.

22

THE DISEASE THAT TURNED OUT
TO BE AIDS

"We live in a world threatened by unlimited destructive force,
yet we share a vision of creative potential . . . AIDS shows us once
again that silence, exclusion, and isolation—of individuals,
groups or nations—creates a danger for us all."

—DR. JONATHAN MANN

IN THE UNITED States, the first cases of the disease that turned out to
be AIDS appeared in the mid-1970s. There had been sporadic cases of
what was likely the same disease reported throughout the world before
that, but there was never any hint of an epidemic. In the opening stage,
the undiscovered virus responsible for the worldwide spread was primarily
transmitted by sexual activity, through intravenous drug use, and via blood
transfusions. In large measure, the spread of the virus occurred globally
because the 1970s represented the first generation of large numbers of
international and intercontinental airline travelers.

How did the epidemic start? No one is sure about its origins, which were in Africa. But by the late 1970s, some formerly rare diseases were proliferating in urban areas of the United States. There seemed to be no obvious connection between the outbreaks of these unusual pulmonary conditions, neurologic illnesses, and skin diseases. But what was becoming apparent was that these unusual diseases were showing up disproportionately in discrete groups of people: drug users, hemophiliacs, and homosexuals.

So although the HIV virus was not formally identified until 1983, the AIDS epidemic is considered to have actually begun a half decade earlier. Of course, at the time, nobody knew these were AIDS patients; no one knew what an AIDS patient was. It wasn't until the early 1980s that the diagnostic patterns began to take shape.

There were three primary epicenters of the United States where large numbers of these patients were being seen: San Francisco, primarily at San Francisco General Hospital; New York, primarily at St. Vincent's Hospital (where I'd interviewed as a medical student); and Chicago, at Cook County. I started my residency at County just as the first AIDS patients were showing up.

All these years later, I still remember our first cases, all of which occurred in 1977. It was only after nearly a decade of hindsight that it became obvious that these three cases were related. They were certainly among the first AIDS cases in Chicago, and probably among the earliest in the United States.

————————

I was on call with one of my fellow residents, and he admitted a patient with a condition none of us had ever seen before. The patient was a twenty-three-year-old man who had strange blotchy, purple skin lesions on his arms and chest. His only medical history, which seemed unrelated, was that he had recently been treated for venereal disease in one of the city's satellite clinics. A fact that didn't appear to be relevant then, but in retrospect probably was significant, was that the satellite clinic was in the Broadway/Belmont area—a.k.a. Boystown, at the time Chicago's principal gay neighborhood.

The resident presenting the case at our morning conference the next day was quite experienced, having done some training in Europe before coming to the United States. Part of his training had included spending time in dermatology, which turned out to be fortunate, because he identified the lesions as resembling Kaposi's sarcoma, an extremely rare malignant skin tumor. Most of the room had never heard of Kaposi's sarcoma, much less seen it. The disease was first described in 1872 by a European physician, Morris Kaposi, in men in their fifties and sixties:

> Nodules the size of shot, peas, or hazelnuts and brown-red to blue-red in color develop in the skin without a known general or local cause. Their surface is smooth, their consistency coarse-elastic; they sometimes swell like an angioma. They are either isolated and then protrude, after becoming larger, in a spherical shape, or else they form groups and remain flatter. . . . They ordinarily appear first on the sole of the foot and the instep, and not long afterwards, also on the hands. The largest numbers generally develop on these parts of the body, where they are accompanied by diffuse thickening of the skin and deformation of the hands and feet . . .

Fortunately, an experienced staff dermatologist came into the conference to discuss the case with us. He acknowledged that the description of the lesions the resident provided resembled Kaposi's sarcoma, but he couldn't believe it. Kaposi's sarcoma was virtually unheard of in such a young man. Even he had only seen a few cases in his forty-year career, and those conformed to the classical age distribution of a much older population.

He was anxious to go to the patient's bedside and look at the lesions. Once there, he was stunned; this was most likely Kaposi's sarcoma in a twenty-three-year-old, an excellent diagnosis by the resident. He opined that once the patient had a biopsy, which quickly confirmed the diagnosis, the case was so rare that the resident should write it up as a case report in a medical journal.

The resident was never able to prepare a case report, because he was so busy with his clinical duties and probably thought this was an anomaly that would quickly be forgotten. But in less than a year, extremely unusual cases of Kaposi's sarcoma like the one this young man had were being reported all over the country.

We started seeing more cases like it. Oddly enough, almost all of them seemed to come from young men from the Broadway/Belmont neighborhood. And we couldn't figure out why.

———————

A month after this, another young man came into the intensive care unit with severe shortness of breath. His only known medical history was that he was an intravenous drug user. His X-ray revealed a severe pneumonia. The pneumonia had an atypical pattern, and our initial thought was that he had a heart valve infection from injecting drugs, which had seeded his lungs. But all the cultures of his blood were negative.

His pneumonia got worse and his condition deteriorated; we gave him our strongest antibiotics but they seemed to have no effect. Soon he was not able to get enough oxygen into his lungs, and he required a breathing tube and ventilator to keep breathing. The pneumonia continued to worsen. Our pulmonary doctors decided to do a bronchoscopy, a procedure in which a scope is inserted through the breathing tube into the lungs to obtain some lung tissue and sample it for cultures. To our shock, the culture came back with an extremely rare organism called *Pneumocystis*. It was not even a bacterium; it was more like a fungus.

This explained why our antibiotics were not working: they were for bacteria, and therefore were not effective against this organism. But nothing else was clear. What was going on?

Pneumocystis was occasionally observed in newborns and in cancer patients whose immune systems had been weakened by chemotherapy. Our patient was an otherwise healthy twenty-five-year-old. It made no sense that this organism should be proliferating in his lungs.

By coincidence that day, we had a visiting professor, one of the country's top infectious disease doctors, from Stanford. If anyone would have the answer to the puzzle of this young man with a rare pneumonia, he would. We presented the case to him in a special conference.

After hearing the presentation the infectious disease expert shrugged; he had no better idea than we did as to why this patient should have pneumonia caused by *Pneumocystis*. That in itself was unusual, since infectious disease experts almost always have a theory about rare cases. He said that in twenty-plus years of treating infectious disease, all his cases of *Pneumocystis* were in patients with weakened immune systems. Yet there was no evidence this patient had a weakened immune system.

The drug user in our ICU died the next day. No one connected him to the young man with Kaposi's sarcoma, nor was there reason to do so. They were both in their twenties, but that was their only similarity. The drug user was black, with rare acute pulmonary disease. He lived on the South Side of Chicago. The young man with Kaposi's sarcoma was white, from the North Side of the city. They were both patients at our hospital, but other than that, they had nothing in common. Or so we thought back then.

However, the Stanford expert made a brief mention of one interesting thing that we realized later might have been a clue. Apparently one of his infectious disease colleagues in California had recently seen several young, healthy men die of severe pneumonia. In the absence of an influenza epidemic, it was strange for young men to die of pneumonia and there was no such influenza epidemic going on at the time. He told us these young men had died in San Francisco.

It wasn't long after this that we were confronted with another puzzle in the ICU. A young man was admitted with a neurologic problem that, again, we were not able to diagnose. The patient was confused, then progressed to lethargy, and finally wound up comatose. He received every diagnostic test we had, but none of the results were conclusive, though many were abnormal. His spinal tap suggested he had an infection that resembled encephalitis, but no infection could be cultured.

We ordered a CT scan, which at that time was not routine; we had to send him across the street to another hospital to obtain one (and more than one unstable patient had died at night during those trips to the outside CT scanner in the early years). When the patient finally did receive a CT scan, the radiologist pronounced the results different from anything he had ever seen.

The patient kept deteriorating while consultant after consultant was called in. As so often happens, each specialty had its own idea about what was wrong. A specialist is like a kid with a hammer—everything is a nail. But no one had the answer to what was wrong with the patient.

Ultimately, the patient died—of a mysterious undiagnosed neurologic disease. Another clue that was, unfortunately, ignored: he was a recent immigrant from Haiti. But that seemed at the time to be of no significance.

So in a brief span of time in 1977, three mystery patients were admitted: a young man with Kaposi's sarcoma, who may have been gay; an intravenous drug user with *Pneumocystis* pneumonia; and a Haitian immigrant with something that may have been encephalitis. No one knew it then, but it now seems almost certain that they all had AIDS.

A decade later, when I put the pieces of the long-ago puzzle together and realized that these were all AIDS patients, I marveled at how fortunate we were. In the 1970s, we rarely wore gloves when drawing blood, putting in intravenous lines, or examining patients. We didn't cap needles, and took a completely casual attitude to being drenched in a patient's blood during resuscitation: *Go home, wash it off.*

Doctors and nurses are at a serious risk when they treat patients with infectious disease—as evidenced during the recent Ebola outbreak. This will be a more common problem for health care workers in the future. Even in those days, we knew there was a risk of blood-borne hepatitis from patients' blood. Yet despite contact with those three patients who probably harbored HIV (and likely others before we knew about the virus), no one who treated them became infected. I shudder when I remember that I had the Haitian patient's blood all over my arms several times. Had I or anyone else become infected from their blood, it would have been a death sentence in those days.

Lucky.

When HIV was identified in 1983, there was a great deal of controversy between the French and the Americans over who first isolated the virus. Regardless, by 1985 the world knew about AIDS; the height of the epidemic, at least in the United States, occurred over the next decade and a half. Cook County was treating more AIDS patients than any hospital outside the East and West Coasts.

During the early days of the epidemic, some doctors refused to take care of AIDS patients and some intensive care units refused to admit them, believing that there was no point—that is, that they would all die anyway. At County we were determined to care for them, and our ICU probably took care of as many AIDS patients as any in North America, possibly in the world. The most common condition that brought these patients to the ICU was *Pneumocystis* pneumonia. Of course, I recalled the first case I ever saw, before there was AIDS.

I was interviewed in 1994 for a book about County called *Hospital*, by Sydney Lewis. I recounted what was the most difficult administrative decision I ever made concerning AIDS patients with pneumonia:

Back in '86 we lost our first, roughly, ten AIDS patients who were in Intensive Care. One of the AIDS social workers . . . felt we should do hospice. Her argument was based on compassion: she didn't want to see all these people suffer . . . yet it was unprecedented, in my experience, to have a specific disease where you say that just because they have this disease, you don't put them in Intensive Care. About three months later we had a survivor. Well, the moment you have one survivor, you now turn it into a much more complicated ethical question.

Within a year, we began to see more and more survivors. We began to develop certain patterns, we were learning how to do things. In the late 1980's we published our first paper on it, saying the mortality of this disease in the ICU is not 80 to 90%, it's actually 50 to 60% . . . We were vilified. Every reviewer said, "You gotta be making this up, this isn't our experience." But what was a big issue five or six years ago is not even a question today: nobody thinks twice about admitting an AIDS patient to the unit today. That is a radical change from a long time ago . . . The field can change very quickly.

The field did change very quickly. Within a few years, there were prophylactic antibiotics that would prevent *Pneumocystis* pneumonia. Then came antiretroviral drugs, which can render the AIDS virus quiescent for years. Today, there are very few AIDS patients with *Pneumocystis* in the ICU, because the virus's immunosuppressive effects are so well controlled. There is no cure yet, but hopefully that day will come soon. We are so much closer than we were in those early days.

The scope of the epidemic changed with the advent of antiretroviral drugs in the twenty-first century. The story of AIDS in the 1970s and '80s was one of pessimism. Today it is one of optimism.

23

CHICAGO HAS TWO SEASONS

"Chicago is the coldest place on earth where
polar bears don't roam free."

—LEWIS GRIZZARD

AFTER HIS FIRST winter in Chicago, the Southern humorist Lewis Grizzard could be excused for indulging in a slight bit of overstatement—among major American cities, Anchorage, Milwaukee, Madison, and Minneapolis are all colder than Chicago—but the Chicago cold is legend. It is the coldest large city and the largest cold city in the United States. When it whips off Lake Michigan, the wind, a.k.a. "the Hawk," creates a windchill that sends a message to even the hardiest soul. (The great Chicago jazz/blues singer Lou Rawls did a wonderfully descriptive opening monologue on "the Hawk" on his classic 1967 recording "Dead End Street.") For doctors working in an ICU in Chicago, it means taking care of people who suffer from the ravages of exposure—in the case of cold, hypothermia.

Chicago is a cold weather city, and hypothermia (below-normal body temperature) is a far more common reason for admission to the ICU than hyperthermia (extreme excess body heat). For one thing, the body adjusts to hot weather more quickly than it does to cold. In the era of air-conditioning, it is far easier for people to survive the extremes of summer than of winter. While a couple of hours outside in subzero cold without appropriate clothing may be fatal, most people can withstand the worst heat of summer for longer periods. No one is likely to suffer hyperthermia from roaming aimlessly for an hour or so in the heat, unless they are in Death Valley or the Sahara.

But in the winter months, people who were outside for long periods of time and could not find shelter often came to the hospital with hypothermia. It was also not unusual to have old people present with low body temperatures because their homes or apartments were not heated adequately. In general, the elderly do not tolerate even a moderately cold environment well, and the old who are also poor are at special risk.

Alcoholics who made it to the hospital after wandering outside in the cold were the lucky ones. Many others died before ever reaching it; a single ill-advised or inebriated decision often proved fatal. In a tragic cautionary tale, Teresa McGovern, the daughter of senator and 1972 presidential candidate George McGovern, was found lifeless in a snowbank. She had been outside for only a few hours after an alcohol binge during a harsh winter in Madison, Wisconsin. Every year the newspapers will carry a story of a child who wanders out of the house in the winter; rescuers often have only minutes to find the child, depending on the temperature outside, because children have even less tolerance for cold.

The danger of cold water is another thing most people don't appreciate. During the winter, patients would be brought to the hospital with immersion hypothermia after being rescued from the Chicago River or Lake Michigan following a drinking binge or a suicide attempt. But most people pulled from the water were not brought to the ICU—they were DOA. The body loses heat much faster in water than it does in air, so a winter plunge into cold water will kill you unless you are rescued almost immediately.

The same thing can and does happen in the summer, albeit more slowly. Unless they are in the warm waters of the tropics, people who fall off a boat, or who decide to leave the boat and go swimming, may become hypothermic. Anyone who goes on a summer swim knows the risks. If the water is warm enough and the time in the water is short enough, the swimmer merely suffers a chill. Getting out of the water and being rewarmed by the sun restores body temperature quickly. But even in warm water—say, 75°F—being immersed for a long enough duration means the body loses heat and death is possible. It takes only a matter of hours. Even experienced swimmers die in boating accidents when help does not arrive quickly enough.

During a winter cold snap, hypothermic patients often came to the hospital in bunches. Sometimes a late autumn cold front that suddenly drops the temperature from 55°F to 25°F in a half day will catch homeless people by surprise. The same thing happens to hunters, mountain climbers, and hikers who get caught in a quick change in the weather and are not prepared for a sudden drop in the temperature. A person with a body temperature below 90°F would generally be admitted to our ICU for rewarming. Most of those patients could be warmed quickly and suffered no lasting effects, unless they had underlying diseases or happened to contract infections like pneumonia.

In a typical Chicago winter, fatal hypothermia was more common at body temperatures below 85°F. The lower the temperature drops below 85°F, the less likely the patient is to survive.

Especially frustrating was the occasional case of a patient who was alive but very cold when admitted to the hospital and who then died during rewarming, unable to be resuscitated. This is presumably because the body's core continues to cool for a brief time even after the body has started to rewarm. Those people are right on the edge—their hearts cannot tolerate even a brief continuing temperature drop. This happens commonly in shipwrecks: survivors are rescued from the cold water and are rewarming but then die a short time afterward.

The coldest patient we ever rescued had a body temperature of 73°F. She was a young alcoholic woman with a strong heart who, like Teresa McGovern, happened to venture from a tavern out into the cold, and she was without a coat. The police found her rather quickly and brought her to us. She had no measurable blood pressure and barely had a heartbeat. Fortunately, she rewarmed quickly and within three days, she was ready to leave the ICU. For all intents and purposes, she was clinically dead when brought in. Some of the staff considered it a miracle (but it should be noted that the lowest reported body temperature for a few survivors is far lower, in the high 50s).

No matter what anyone says, it is not just medical skill; luck plays a huge part in these cases. Unlike Teresa McGovern, this particular girl was fortunate that she had been found quickly, and that she responded to rewarming and didn't suffer any complications. Fate was on her side; it could easily have gone the other way. In cases like hers that are reported in medical journals and newspapers where there is a fine line between life and death, the doctors rarely mention the role of luck. But luck is important.

To her credit, after that close encounter with death, this young woman said she would swear off alcohol. I did see her once or twice in the clinic after that, and she had indeed given up drinking. You only get so many warnings, and she heeded hers.

——————————

There is an adage in emergency and intensive care medicine: *no one is dead until they are warm and dead*. It means that hypothermic patients may appear to be dead but they should not be declared dead until an attempt has been made to rewarm them. An illustrative case from Britain in the 2002 *Emergency Medicine Journal* about a man whose temperature was 63°F (17°C):

A 37 year old man was found in his garden cold with no signs of life. Pupils were fixed and dilated. Electrocardiography showed asystole initially. The paramedic crew started cardiopulmonary resuscitation and transferred him to the accident and emergency department. His temperature was 17.0°C. Cardiopulmonary resuscitation was continued for three hours before rewarming using partial cardiopulmonary bypass. He eventually regained spontaneous cardiac output and made a full neurological recovery. Hypothermic patients with no evidence of life cannot be assumed to be dead as there is a chance of full recovery when fully warmed.

Such is the dilemma in cases like this. This man easily could have been called DOA when he came to the hospital. If a hypothermic patient comes in without a pulse, when should we attempt to rewarm him and when should we declare him dead? No doubt many hours of effort have been expended attempting to rewarm patients who are truly dead. I never resolved this issue completely to my satisfaction.

We once had a young woman who was admitted with a body temperature of 77°F and a barely palpable pulse. She was not unlike our patient who had survived at 73°F, but this patient's heart stopped as we tried to rewarm her with warm blankets, saline, and oxygen. If there was ever a case of "not dead until warm and dead," this was it. For a while she had no blood pressure but a faint electrocardiogram tracing. We worked frantically, attempting every monitoring and therapeutic technique, except for cardiopulmonary bypass (CPB), the technique that was used on the British patient. This method employs machinery that removes all the blood from the body, rewarms it, and provides it with oxygen when the heart is not beating—it essentially bypasses the heart.

At County, we never had access to that most aggressive form of rewarming. For more than a decade, I lobbied for access to this technique. It was available in the hospital but never used outside the operating room, and despite my protestations, no one ever took the initiative to allow its use for rewarming. If there was ever a patient whose life might have been saved with this technique, it was she. I silently cursed the doctors and administrators who refused to let us use CPB for rewarming as we struggled to resuscitate her. For three hours we worked on trying to rewarm her, but it was virtually impossible since her blood was not circulating. At some point in the middle of the resuscitation, her electrocardiogram showed a flat line, but we continued.

For at least an hour and a half, we could not say whether she was alive or dead since we could not raise her temperature. Even today, I do not know the answer to that question; in cases of extreme hypothermia even doctors can't tell the difference between life and death. Ultimately, we were unable to rewarm her, and I had no option but to declare her dead. I am still haunted by that.

––––––––––––

My colleagues and I were faced with a similar issue if we happened to be working in the emergency room when a police wagon—called a squadrol—came to the hospital with a dead body. Police rules required that a doctor had to declare the person dead. So a doctor would get called from the emergency room to go to the parking lot outside the hospital. The doctor would have to climb into the back of the wagon, where there was a dead body, usually an alcoholic from Skid Row, and just say, "Yep, the guy is dead."

The problem came when there was no way of telling for certain whether the person in the squadrol was actually dead. Sometimes it was obvious— massive head trauma, a bullet wound in the heart, or evidence of rigor mortis—but most of them were just bodies lying there with no external marks. The lighting was bad, especially at night, and there was really no way to conduct an examination. Some doctors would actually listen to the chest, but no one ever heard anything and I'm not sure how reliable that was, considering the circumstances. The police, with better things to do, understandably did not want us taking the body out of the van for an electrocardiogram, and the nurses wanted that even less.

Of course, the issue of "not dead until warm and dead" never came up; it would have been completely impractical. So it was just up to us to look at the body and pronounce death. We did it, and we were perpetually uncomfortable about it. Over coffee we often wondered if we had ever made a mistake. Had someone who was pronounced dead actually woken up in the morgue? We never heard about anyone who did. But it could have happened (and in the occasional report it *has* happened), and for fear of a mistake, no one wanted to be the senior physician when two police officers came through the emergency room and said, "Doc, we need you outside to pronounce a stiff in our squadrol." Shades of Edgar Allan Poe's "The Premature Burial."

———————

January may be the cruelest month in Chicago, but as another saying goes, "Chicago has two seasons: winter and construction." Most of the infamous road construction happens in the summer, and at that time of year the city can be sweltering. The temperature in Chicago routinely drops below zero in the winter, but it is not unusual for it to climb above 100°F in the summer. So the same ICU team that must be adept at warming hypothermic patients in the winter also needs to be adept at cooling hyperthermic patients in the summer.

The human body has developed protective mechanisms, like perspiring, to guard against overheating. That's why we can remain outside longer in the heat than in the cold. It's probably an evolutionary adaptation to the fact that man has existed in warm environments longer than we have lived in cold ones. But once those mechanisms are breached, the person does not tolerate a rise in body temperature as well as it does a drop. Patients often survive a deviation of 13° below normal at temperatures of 85°F, but death is almost certain at 112°F, an equivalent deviation of 13° above normal.

Hyperthermia is not simply a high body temperature. Many patients with a wide variety of illnesses run fevers that go up to, and occasionally over, 105°F. That is generally a normal physiologic response and can be protective in fighting infection. However, once the body temperature reaches 106°F, it is usually not a fever; it means the patient has entered a danger zone of excess body heat. The majority of cases of hyperthermia today are due to medication reactions or an adverse response to anesthesia. However, in the face of severe heat waves, people who have been in a hot environment too long can develop life-threatening hyperthermia, commonly known as heatstroke.

Whatever the specialty, when doctors get together, it's not uncommon for the bragging to start about extreme lab values or conditions they have seen. If it's laboratory values, it might be the highest blood sugar or the highest blood sodium concentration you've seen. The closest analogy I can make is basketball players sitting around comparing the most points they ever scored in a game.

When reading the medical literature, to compare with their experience doctors often look for "record values." Every so often, you may think you have seen a record that could make it into the literature with a case report. However, you may be shot down by journal editors who, like the editors at Guinness World Records, inform you that, sorry, yours is not a record—but thanks for trying.

The most severe case of hyperthermia we ever had in the ICU was during the infamous heat wave of 1995, when a man presented with a rectal temperature of 111°F. It was the middle of July, he was a roofer, and his high body temperature was due to working in a daytime temperature over 100°F, standing on a black tar roof that absorbed the heat. Under those conditions, he might have been working in a local environment where the temperature was equivalent to 140°F for several hours. In a situation like this, the body starts to accumulate heat faster than it can dissipate it. People generally can't tolerate a body temperature rise to over 110°F; at that point, the high temperature begins to unravel the proteins of the body, causing brain and liver damage.

With prompt cooling and a great job by the nurses and residents, this patient survived, without brain damage. It is certainly not the highest temperature at which survival has been recorded—that is in the range of 115°F—but this case was impressive. He easily could have died; like the girl with hypothermia who survived after wandering in the cold, he was lucky. Again, fate was on his side as well.

With the exception of the ICUs and the operating rooms, County Hospital then was not air-conditioned. During that 1995 heat wave, the indoor temperature was stifling and the hospital environment itself became unsafe. The heat severely affected some patients whose medications or conditions made it difficult for their bodies to dissipate heat. Some of these people came to the ICU or died because they actually suffered heatstroke *while they were patients in the hospital.*

In a national bestseller, a prominent author described how, during the 1995 heat wave, a heroic County doctor (one of my superiors at the time) marched an administrator onto the oppressively hot ward in an attempt to get portable air conditioners. It made for a good story, made the protagonists look good, but I remember the episode a little differently. As the doctor responsible for monitoring the situation, I made personal entreaties, but there were two heatstroke deaths in the hospital and several ICU admissions for hyperthermia before anyone considered installing air conditioners. No one did anything for days while patients sweltered. So by my account, there was more administrative torpor, and neither the doctor nor the story was quite as heroic as portrayed in the bestseller.

It seems incredible today that people would die of heatstroke in the hospital. But a decade later—in New Orleans, in the aftermath of Hurricane Katrina—patients died of hyperthermia when the hospital lost all power in the sweltering heat. Administrative torpor may have played a role there as well, but in any event, luck works both ways.

24

WORKING IN A FREE CLINIC: HEALTH WITHOUT WEALTH

"The deed is everything, the glory naught."

—GOETHE

WITH THE CONSOLIDATION of the health care industry, many of America's academic medical centers, hospitals, and clinics have become high-tech. This has been a mixed blessing, because while most deliver better care than ever before, budgets commonly escalate from millions to billions, requiring the institutions that deliver health care to redefine their missions. Unlike in the past, today's hospitals and clinics, both in the for-profit and the not-for-profit sector, depend on the free market. While these institutions still provide some charitable care, it is usually a small percentage of their budgets. Their social service functions and local obligations have, in many cases, become subordinated to other imperatives, such as the requirement to raise money and provide jobs for the community, as well as the need to cultivate political influence and community prestige.

It was not always this way. Before World War II, most hospitals and clinics were not expected to support themselves. A century ago, when medicine was less sophisticated, the wealthy often received care in their homes, while the middle class and poor were often cared for in hospitals for extended periods. Sometimes these patients were hospitalized for social reasons, and it was understood that they would not always be able to pay their bills. In the 1920s, only about one-half of patients actually paid for their services, with philanthropy and government making up the difference.

The situation changed forever after World War II, when employers began providing health insurance as a workplace benefit to their employees. An acceleration of this trend occurred in the 1960s as the federal government ramped up medical spending with the Medicare program. Another impetus came in the 1980s when hospitals and clinics began turning to private financing for new construction and expansion. In the 2000s, a wave of mergers and consolidations in the hospital sector rendered the stand-alone community hospital a virtual relic of the past.

Today, there remains one vestige of the simpler, earlier era: the free community clinic. Many of these clinics were set up in urban areas in the 1960s and '70s to provide free outpatient medical care to anyone, no questions asked. Staffed primarily by health care volunteers and a few salaried employees, they received whatever funding they could get from local governments, religious orders, or charitable donations. They served the uninsured by providing medical care and social services, in some cases working in tandem with community hospitals and clinics. (The quintessential 1960s free clinic was portrayed in the 1969 film *Change of Habit*, a "guilty pleasure" starring Elvis Presley as a doctor working in a free clinic and Mary Tyler Moore as his nurse assistant who happens to be a nun.) Though many of these free clinics fell by the wayside—victims of insufficient funding—some have survived and even thrived. A new generation of clinics sprang up in the 1980s and '90s with better funding and more staffing, but with the same mission: to serve the poor and uninsured.

I worked in two free clinics at the bookends of my career. When I was just out of training in the early 1980s, I moonlighted at the Free Medical Clinic of Greater Cleveland. (Established in 1970 as a telephone hotline, it is currently the second oldest and one of the largest free clinics in the United States. In a stark reflection of the inequality of American medical care, the free clinic is located only a short distance from two of the country's most wealthy and prestigious medical centers.) When I retired, my career came full circle, and I worked at a free clinic in Chicago that provides medical, dental, and eye care on the North Side of the city.

Over the past three decades, medicine and medical care have changed remarkably; working in a hospital today is nothing like it was in 1980. But working at a free clinic remains largely unchanged from the past: the experiences and the challenges it provides, the obstacles and difficulties faced, and the support, volunteers, services, and supplies that are always needed.

The most gratifying thing about working at a free clinic is the sense of accomplishment and the spirit of camaraderie that comes from working with other people—such as nurses, pharmacists, and secretaries—who are there to help patients. These patients really need assistance; usually they have nowhere to go and no one else to turn to. Patients exhibit genuine gratitude for what is done for them, even in situations in which their problems, medical or otherwise, are unsolvable with the resources available. Occasionally, a patient may grumble or complain—these are, after all, people who have had a rough go at life—but without question, their level of appreciation for everyone working in a free clinic is greater than in any other medical setting in which I have ever worked. This, in turn, creates a special esprit de corps among those who work at the clinic that is probably akin to that seen in the military: everyone working together for a common purpose, subordinating their own interests to a shared goal.

The exhilaration is contagious. As with the patients, it is unusual to hear the staff complain. In a hospital or a regular clinic, there is often some personal animosity just beneath the surface, a tension caused by a staff member who resents something or someone. You just don't often see that attitude at a free clinic. When I initially started working at the Free Clinic of Cleveland, I was assigned Monday nights. This was in the early 1980s, when watching Monday Night Football on television with friends was a weekly ritual. My assignment meant I couldn't be there for the weekly party. At first, I was annoyed and actually thought about giving up the idea of working there. But after a few weeks, the experience in the clinic was so enjoyable, I didn't miss the football game or the weekly party at all. It was a therapeutic experience—for me.

————————

Most free clinic patients have some combination of the following characteristics: poor, uninsured, unemployed, homeless, lacking English skills, no history of preventive medical care, chronic health problems (especially diabetes and hypertension), psychiatric conditions, drug and/or alcohol problems, and little or no family support. Even the most skilled practitioner would be challenged in this setting, and the first challenge is the necessity to remain nonjudgmental.

The fact that most patients are sick and in need of a significant level of medical attention, nursing care, and follow-up is one of the inherent difficulties. Patients with multiple medical conditions require extensive testing and observation, which means they must come to the clinic frequently. Often this is a barrier, especially if they have to travel a long way on public transportation. Some don't have mailing addresses or telephones, making continuity of care problematic. Patients with multiple medical problems usually need many medications. This is further complicated when patients have trouble adhering to medication schedules or experience debilitating drug side effects or interactions.

Not all free clinic patients come from underprivileged backgrounds; a surprising number are the victims of recent misfortune. Some are middle- and upper-class patients who have lost their jobs and health insurance. Other patients come as a result of a messy divorce or the death of a spouse;

the free clinic often sees widows who live alone and have no way of getting their medications. Occasionally there are patients who were once stock traders or executives or had positions at white-shoe law firms. They had received their medical care in the toniest clinics of the Upper West Side of Manhattan, Chicago's Gold Coast, or West L.A., but once they lost their jobs, their problems were often the same as those of the homeless.

In a regular clinic practice, it's disappointing to see your relationship with patients end after the two of you have forged a bond over time; they come in and tell you they won't be seeing you anymore because they are moving, or they have found a more convenient clinic, or their insurance coverage has changed. Yet in a free clinic, that is the best news you can get. There is nothing better than hearing a patient say, "I liked having you as a doctor, but I found a job with health insurance and I won't be coming back anymore." It's like having a child graduate from college and leave home—your sadness in seeing them leave is trivial compared to the pride and happiness you feel for them.

Resources, resources, resources. Every free clinic is in need of more. Physician specialists needed for consultations are often the hardest thing to find. There is a constant need for surgeons, orthopedists, gynecologists, cardiologists, gastroenterologists, urologists, endocrinologists, dermatologists, and psychiatrists, among others. When there is no specialist available, there is often no alternative but to send the patient to a local emergency room—an expensive, inefficient approach.

For the doctors who work at the free clinic, the lack of specialists and their expertise is also frustrating in subtler ways. At the clinic where I worked, we noticed a pattern of a benign but unusual liver condition in many of the patients who were Russian immigrants. The condition did not adversely affect their health, and it may have been a coincidence, but if not, it suggests a genetic predisposition in that population, something not described in the medical literature. Though it's an interesting hypothesis, it is not likely to be tested, simply because the resources and personnel are not available. Little things like that make you miss the advantages of the major medical center.

Free clinics rely on volunteer services—not just nurses, doctors, and specialty practitioners but also dentists, podiatrists, mental health workers, physical therapists, dieticians, and health educators. Sometimes occupational or legal advice may be needed. In clinics with large immigrant populations, translators are often in short supply. A free clinic is an excellent place for bilingual high school and college students to obtain entry-level volunteer experience. The general public can also play a role, perhaps through the donation of a computer, a television set, or even magazines for the waiting room.

Also commonly in short supply are testing equipment, bandages, and instruments for minor surgery. A free clinic without access to medication is not a clinic. Many medications are expensive and hard to come by, and patients often need help enrolling in patient assistance programs. The large pharmaceutical companies have a role in donating medications to keep free clinic pharmacies stocked. Medical professionals, medical schools, and hospitals can donate excess medical supplies, equipment, and educational materials.

In one treatment room where I worked, someone had generously donated some medical textbooks as references. Unfortunately, a 1946 edition of *Common Surgical Problems* or a 1949 copy of *Gynecology for the General Practitioner* was of little help.

With the growing economic inequality and a surge in immigration, more American families face unprecedented economic pressures. Many people, perhaps even a friend or neighbor of yours, may be only one paycheck away from being without health insurance, a job, and in some cases even a place to live. Hospitals and private clinics, with an eye toward the bottom line, may be unwilling or unable to care for those living so precariously. When such people get sick, require counseling, or simply need medication, free clinics may be their only salvation.

The general public will always need the services of free clinics, and at the same time money, volunteer services, and supplies are part and parcel of what free clinics always need most: the support of the general public.

25

YOU CAN'T STOP PROGRESS

"We are all just prisoners here, of our own device."
—The Eagles, "Hotel California"

THE FORTY-YEAR SPAN of the events in this book roughly equates to the length of a typical medical career. From a scientific perspective, the changes in medicine since the 1970s have ushered in a veritable golden age for patients. Organ transplantation, biopharmacology, MRI and PET scanners, robotics, the Internet, and other innovations afford patients diagnostic modalities and treatments undreamed of four decades ago. Unquestionably, most patients live longer, better lives (at least those who don't die of hospital-acquired infections or complications from unnecessary testing). And while antibiotics, which came to the fore after World War II, have seen their effectiveness diminish as a result of increased resistance, on the whole it is hard to find fault with the benefits of modern medicine.

From the standpoint of the jobs they are tasked with, things have improved for health care professionals as well. Once, doctors had to draw blood and perform ECGs on patients by themselves, something today's doctors and patients have only heard about in books like this. Today, there are whole departments of technicians to do those tasks. Likewise, nurses have been relieved of much of their physical work by aides and assistants. Computers are ubiquitous on the wards; a pen is hard to find and pencils have essentially vanished. Even the term "hospital" is gradually disappearing—multimillion-dollar medical centers, and even community hospitals, are now increasingly referred to as "campuses," an inflated term that confers a modicum of academic respectability, whether deserved or not.

Compared to how it was forty years ago, what's not to like about medicine today?

The answer lies in one word: *depersonalization*. At heart, medicine is about people's personalities and emotions—their insecurities, fears, frailties, and the like. Not just those of patients but also those of doctors, nurses, and other health care workers. To an extent, that was the reason for this book: to portray some of those personalities for the reader from the perspective of my decades in the profession.

From every angle, medicine is becoming more depersonalized than ever before. Though it is by no means a new trend—physicians have been depersonalizing patients since the days of Hippocrates—it is simply more sophisticated today. Yet it remains antithetical to the best traditions of medicine. The trend is evident all around us, whether it is the computer screen that discourages eye contact with the patient, the technicians who make it unnecessary for the doctor and nurse to touch the patient, or just the new bureaucratic jargon that turns the hospital into the medical center or campus. (Imagine someone saying, "Mom, Dad isn't feeling well. I think we should take him over to the medical center campus.")

The patient has become a depersonalized entity, and despite all the high-tech and sophisticated medical care, this loss of identity does not bode well for any of us who will be patients in the future, which means pretty much all of us.

Moreover, despite the former prestige associated with being a doctor, many—even the younger ones—are now considering leaving the profession. And there is greater impetus to do so than ever before, with the well-documented loss of autonomy, the spate of bureaucratic rules foisted on the profession by the government and third-party payers, and faux improvements in medical practice like the electronic medical record, which promises much and delivers little. Combine all that with the growing specialization in health care, and the days of having a longtime family doctor or personal doctor are mostly over. It is unlikely today's doctors will stay in the profession as long as those who practiced fifty or a hundred years ago. Experience, and the knowledge that comes with it, are being lost.

How did all this happen?

Two critical paradigm shifts.

The two underlying but unstated themes of this book were first, that doctors had a *covenant* relationship with patients, and second, that health care was supposed to operate along the *virtue* model—not that it always did, but it was supposed to. Today, the covenant relationship between doctor and patient is being replaced by a *contractual* relationship, and the virtue model of health care is being replaced by the *profit* model.

And "we are all just prisoners here, of our own device."

Covenantal versus contractual: The essence of the covenant between physician and patient was always a common bond, unique and intimate in a way different from friendship or the tie between relatives or lovers. It didn't matter who the patient was—a priest, a prostitute, a gang member, or a policeman. Even a mass murderer or serial killer or terrorist bomber. It didn't matter whether the patient was a healthy hypochondriac or a terminally ill cancer patient. The doctor and the patient had a covenant.

This covenantal relationship was the amalgam of several values including trust, honesty, accountability, availability, and confidentiality. Each generation of doctors was charged with imparting those traits to, and creating that covenant for, the next generation of trainees. But to some degree, the older generation has been derelict in assuming that responsibility and passing it on, so the covenant has been damaged. And it has been further undermined by the bureaucracy that has enveloped medicine.

As an example of what happened, consider *confidentiality*, the familiar covenantal value that expected discussions between patient and doctor to remain private between the two parties. This was a Hippocratic principle: "Whatever, in connection with my professional service, or not in connection with it, I see or hear, in the life of men, which ought not to be spoken of abroad, I will not divulge, as reckoning that all such should be kept secret."

But as part of the changing relationship between doctor and patient, the intrusion of the government subtly changed this principle. In the 1990s, to enforce confidentiality, the government passed HIPAA, the jargon acronym for the Health Insurance Portability and Accountability Act. Passing a law to enforce a centuries-old principle that was theretofore unquestioned was like passing legislation to ensure the army would march in a straight line.

In many ways, for doctors, there was little point in this law. And the law became one of the things—not the only thing, certainly, but one thing— that undermined the covenant by inserting the government between the doctor and patient. Prior to HIPAA, doctors were sometimes lax about confidentiality with their patients, but their transgressions were for the most part minor. Since then, HIPAA has become an enterprise that costs millions of dollars annually and requires armies of personnel to enforce, yet whether confidentiality has improved is questionable. It may well be worse. I have literally seen clergy denied the room numbers of supplicant patients on HIPAA grounds. They are prevented from offering solace because of "confidentiality."

From the doctors' perspective, the minions of enforcement have used the law more as a sword than a shield. Doctors sometimes find it harder to obtain necessary clinical information, while that same information is readily accessible to insurance companies and the government. Combined with the advent of electronic medical records, hackers and miscreants could easily appropriate thousands of confidential records in a few minutes. And they have; the number of hacked medical records is in the millions. And that's just those that have been documented. This would have been unheard of forty years ago. How has the confidential relationship between doctor and patient been served by all of this? Unfortunately, confidentiality is no longer in the hands of the physician. It has become the province of countless others putting themselves between the doctor and patient, and is now couched in forms written in legal language. It is now a *contractual*, rather than a *covenantal* entity. And that is what has happened to the other aspects of the relationship between the doctor and the patient as well.

A contractual relationship does not necessarily mean that the patient and physician have mutually signed a written contract. But today, when physicians and almost everyone else in health care are employed by larger entities, at some point the relationship with patients is indeed drawn up in writing somewhere. Certainly on some level, the connection between physician and patient has been codified, usually in legal terms, and the physician is expected to follow its dictates.

Contracts do not guarantee the aforementioned values of the covenant. A good contract might encourage these values, but those values are no longer essential to the relationship. For example, nowhere does it say, *The physician and the patient should trust each other*, or *should be honest with each other*. Most important, a contractual relationship does not necessarily place as its highest value the benefit of the patient. By definition, a covenant was a common bond, and a contract is a give-and-take of interests. The patient is not necessarily in a higher position.

Which leads to the second theme of *virtue versus profit*. The sine qua non of health care has traditionally been virtue—to help patients, to make them feel better, to save their lives. This raison d'être dates back to Hippocrates and even earlier. Almost all students applying to medical or nursing school submit an essay that talks about their desire to help patients. The explicit virtue model was elaborated on by Aristotle and St. Thomas Aquinas. It was the model on which hospitals were originally based: the desire to heal patients or ameliorate their suffering.

Two of the logical concomitants of the virtue model were the religious affiliations of hospitals and the concept of charity care. For centuries, most hospitals in the United States and Europe were either run by or closely associated with religious entities. It was part of their mission. Similarly, charity care was a critical piece of the hospital function. The threat that uncompensated care posed to the financial well-being of an institution was always present, but it was subordinated in the pursuit of virtue. The hospital that is the subject of so many stories in this book, Cook County, was known and respected as a "charity hospital." Charity was an understood offshoot of virtue.

Even in individual physician/patient interactions, this was true for most of the history of American medicine. When doctors made house calls (now largely a relic of an earlier age), or when patients visited the doctor in his or her office, those who could afford it were expected to pay in cash. The poor, if they could pay at all, would often barter. As many of the stories in this book illustrated, virtue was a powerful motivator in health care.

The great Sir William Osler wrote this of virtue and charity in medicine: "As the practice of medicine is not a business and can never be one, the education of the heart—the moral side of the man—must keep pace with the education of the head. Our fellow creatures cannot be dealt with as man deals in corn and coal; 'the human heart by which we live' must control our professional relations."

That is the philosophy of this book. But no one involved at any level of health care today would argue for very long that virtue, while admittedly still a motivator, is the primary motivator. It has been superseded, at all levels, by the profit motive. It is beyond the scope of this chapter to trace the history of how this occurred or why, but it's safe to say medicine has become a business, and in many cases a ruthless one. Osler's philosophy is dead and buried; our fellow creatures are being dealt with as man deals in corn and coal.

A brief but telling example of this devolution: in older hospitals, portraits of prominent physicians once hung in the hallways for patients and visitors to see. Of course, it was something of an artificial aggrandizement of men who needed no such promotion, but on another level, it did serve as the hospitals' expressions of what they valued: taking care of patients. Today, it is unusual to see those portraits of doctors in older hospitals and even more so in newer ones. Instead there are donor plaques or portraits of the administrators and board members who preside over these institutions.

Another example of how the corporate interest has taken hold: at a community hospital I still visit, a nurse asked me if I was attending the hospital's "corporate loyalty" meeting that afternoon. They were expecting me. I told her, in jest, I was planning on going to the dentist to have a painful root canal procedure and I didn't want to reschedule. I'm sorry, but I didn't go to medical school to attend corporate loyalty meetings.

These examples reveal what is most valued in medicine today: money. To be sure, money always had a prominent role in the practice of medicine. But this book and the stories in it are meant to recall an earlier era when that role was not so prominent. It takes place in another time, when medicine was not as effective as it is today but was more innocent—and more beneficent. The reader can decide which he or she prefers, but it is a moot point, since we can never return to that time and place. As the book of Ecclesiastes says, "What is crooked cannot be made straight, and what is lacking cannot be counted." Contemporary medicine is indeed a crooked place, not necessarily in the sense of being dishonest—though, to be sure, there is some of that. But more important, American medicine today is big business, a maze of profit centers and bureaucracy, a place where "you can check out any time you like, but you can never leave."